Osteoporosis

spending six [...] [...]search. He writes the 'Doctor, Doctor' column in the *Guardian* on Saturdays, and also has columns in the *Bradford Telegraph & Argus*, the *Lancashire Telegraph*, the *Carrick Gazette* and the *Galloway Gazette*. He has written two humorous books, *Doctor, Have You Got a Minute?* and *A Seaside Practice*, both published by Short Books. His other books for Sheldon Press include *Heart Attacks: Prevent and Survive*, *Living with Alzheimer's Disease*, *Coping Successfully with Prostate Cancer*, *Overcoming Back Pain*, *Coping with Bowel Cancer*, *Coping with Heartburn and Reflux*, *Coping with Age-related Memory Loss*, *Skin Cancer: Prevent and Survive*, *How to Get the Best from Your Doctor* and *Coping with Kidney Disease*.

# Overcoming Common Problems Series

*Selected titles*

A full list of titles is available from Sheldon Press,
36 Causton Street, London SW1P 4ST and on our website at
www.sheldonpress.co.uk

# Overcoming Common Problems Series

# Overcoming Common Problems Series

Overcoming Common Problems

# Osteoporosis
## Prevent and treat

DR TOM SMITH

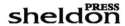

First published in Great Britain in 2008
Sheldon Press
36 Causton Street
London SW1P 4ST

Illustration copyright © Alasdair Smith 2008

*British Library Cataloguing-in-Publication Data*
A catalogue record for this book is available from the British Library

ISBN 978-1-84709-059-1

1 3 5 7 9 10 8 6 4 2

Typeset by Fakenham Photosetting Ltd, Fakenham, Norfolk
Printed in Great Britain by Ashford Colour Press

Produced on paper from sustainable forests

# Contents

# Introduction

You have heard the typical osteoporosis story: 'She fell and broke her hip, and that's when the doctors found she had osteoporosis.' That's not always true. It is quite likely that the person has been walking in the normal way and her thigh bone (femur) has snapped, just at the angle below the joint with the hip bone. *Then* she fell, because her leg had broken, spontaneously.

You can imagine how much strength has been lost out of a thigh bone for it to break in this way. It is the result of many years of loss of bone structure – both minerals and proteins. Why does it often show up first as a fracture near the hip joint? Because that's the part of the skeleton that bears most of our body weight as we walk. There is probably just as much bone structure loss in the arm bones as in the leg, but we don't walk on our hands – we put much less stress through our wrists.

That is, until we slip and fall and put out our hands to break the impact. The result in someone with osteoporosis is a wrist fracture – the second commonest way we find out that a woman has the disease.

The third way is more subtle, and takes longer, mainly because there's no sudden accident to bring the person (again usually a woman) to the doctor. Instead, she has been gradually losing height over several years. She is a bit more stooped than she used to be, and she may have quite a lot of back pain, making it painful to get around. She looks on all these changes as 'being due to her age' and does little about it, except to take painkillers and rest a lot. She gives up most of her physical activities, tending to sit about, rather than expose her weakening frame to exertion.

That creates a vicious circle, in which she takes less exercise, which weakens her bones further, so she takes even less exercise, and so on.

It's only when her doctor sees her, probably for another complaint, that it is recognized for what it is – gradual collapse of her spinal bones (vertebrae) because of osteoporosis. The spine, like the legs, bears a lot of our body weight, and if the bones lose their strength, they crumble. That leads not just to loss of height, but also to pain, due to pressure on the nerves that pass through the gaps between the bones into and out of the spinal cord.

By the time people have arrived at the stage of hip, wrist and vertebral fractures, they are at a very advanced stage of the disease. Their doctors can still help them a lot with modern drugs that shift mineral strength back into their bones, but by this time much of the damage cannot be reversed. We can't give people back their lost height, and broken hips and wrists are often never the same as they were before the fractures. So we need to try to prevent osteoporosis from getting to this crippling stage.

We used to think that the bone loss of osteoporosis started in middle age in both men and women. As men start off with much stronger bones, the loss doesn't become apparent in terms of fractures until 20 years after it starts to take its toll in women. Now we know that, with changing modern lifestyles, many women start to lose bone strength much earlier – it can start in the late teens and early twenties in susceptible women, if they follow the wrong lifestyle. Then, when they lose their monthly hormone surge at the menopause, the bone loss accelerates for a while, so that they lose even more bone for a few years. That puts them at a distinct disadvantage compared with men, and is one reason for osteoporosis being generally thought to be much more of a woman's than a man's illness. That is true to an extent, but older men may also become osteoporotic.

The more we exercise, the stronger our bones get, so that people, particularly women, who exercise regularly can help to keep their bones strong well into old age. They are less likely to develop osteoporosis. But this rule only holds good if you also eat well. If you don't eat, and you exercise purely because you want to become thin, then you can lose bone strength rather than gain it. Women who have had anorexia in their teens and early twenties, and who use excessive exercise to keep their body weight down, are much more likely to develop osteoporosis in later life than those who have retained a normal body shape. Plenty of young women who exercise regularly in gyms are too thin: they are putting themselves at risk for the future if they don't keep up a normal body weight for their height. If you are exercising, don't do it more than five days a week and make sure you eat enough to replace the weight you lose. If you are underweight, you must ask yourself about your motives for exercising, and consider whether what you are doing is ultimately right for you and your long-term health.

Other habits that put you at higher risk of developing osteoporosis include smoking. To the many well-known reasons for avoiding smoke (such as lung, throat, kidney and bladder cancers, chronic lung disease, heart attacks, strokes and limb amputations) must be added osteoporosis. Smokers lose bone density, and the more you smoke, the higher your risk. Other habits that promote osteoporosis include physical inactivity (never exercising at all), drinking too much alcohol and lack of vitamin D.

Vitamin D helps build strong bones, so if we don't eat enough foods containing it (oily fish, butter and eggs are good sources) we can develop osteoporosis. We also make vitamin D in our skin from sunlight, which is the main source of the vitamin in tropical countries. British Asians who wear clothes that cover up their bodies completely are at high risk of vitamin D deficiency, and should make sure that they are getting enough in their diet to counteract their lack of exposure to the sun.

This book is for people with osteoporosis and for those who care for them. It is also for anyone who thinks that they might develop it because of their family history of the illness. It can be avoided or at least postponed for many years, and if it is already established its progress can be slowed and the symptoms greatly alleviated. How this can be achieved is explained in the following pages.

It begins with personal case histories from my own experience in general practice. You may recognize yourself or the person for whom you are caring in one of them. It describes the structure of bones and what happens when they become osteoporotic, and it then explains the way doctors currently manage the illness, from the initial diagnosis and tests to advice on lifestyle and the various modern treatments for it. Happily, there are new, effective treatments for osteoporosis that are proven to strengthen bones and that have been a great help – indeed, a revolution – in the relief of the pain and suffering endured by people with this distressing disease.

There are also controversies about the current treatments – at the time of writing, major new studies of people with osteoporosis challenge the current acceptance of some of today's treatments. They are summarized in Chapter 14.

Despite the trial results, this remains an optimistic book. Its main message is that most people with osteoporosis can still be helped in many ways to ease their symptoms and to strengthen their bones. But it needs your efforts, as well as those of the primary care team of your doctor, nurse and physiotherapist. Above all, it needs your compliance with your modern drug treatment. The trials failed to show a real advantage of treatment mainly because, after a while, the patients failed to keep up with their treatments. After only a year or so, fewer than half of them were still taking their medicines and following the correct lifestyle.

So one aim of this book is to strengthen your resolve to continue to keep up with your various treatments. It is understandable that you may not like the idea of taking tablets and even injections for the rest of your life, or that you really don't want to exercise regularly as you grow older and your bones and muscles ache when you do so. It is particularly difficult to keep on taking your treatment when you get no instant feeling that it is doing you good – in that way it is unlike insulin for diabetes, lack of which soon makes you very ill indeed.

Treating yourself for osteoporosis is more like taking treatment for high blood pressure. You don't feel particularly unwell if you don't take the treatment. But the first symptom that your blood pressure has gone wrong may be a stroke or a heart attack, and when that happens it is too late to start to regret your failure to take your medicines. In the same way, the first symptom of failing to keep up with your osteoporosis treatment may be a hip, wrist or spinal fracture – and they can have consequences that leave you with permanent problems.

There is good evidence that modern management of osteoporosis does prevent or at least postpone fractures for decades. So please read the treatment sections thoroughly and take them to heart. They could save you from a lot of future anguish.

# 1

# People with osteoporosis

*Jane – an older woman*

Jane, at 75, had been unsteady on her feet for several years. She was thin and relatively frail, and tended not to look after herself very well now that she was a widow. Her husband, Herbert, had died three years before, and she was still grieving. She had always been house-proud, but now she felt that there was no-one to be house-proud for, so she hadn't bothered to change her threadbare carpets, preferring to place the odd rug down over the bits of wear and tear.

She was struggling, too, to manage her money, now that she was surviving on a low pension, so she tended to cut corners that would never have been cut when Herbert was alive. She didn't eat as well as she should, preferring a sandwich to the bother of making meals. And her teeth didn't fit so well, so that she rarely ate anything that needed biting and chewing, like fruit and vegetables. Neighbours tried to persuade her to take meals-on-wheels, but she saw that as charity and her pride didn't let her accept it. There was an element, too, of not wanting to let outsiders see the state she was in.

So it was inevitable that one day Jane tripped over the edge of one of her rugs, and fell sideways on to her left hip. She knew it had gone as it happened. She heard the snap of the bone. It wasn't particularly painful, but when she tried to rise, she couldn't put weight on her leg. She dragged herself to the phone and called the emergency services. The ambulance came in minutes, and she was in hospital and having treatment within hours. She was given a replacement hip joint and within a couple of weeks was back at home, but this time with a full care team to support her, including people to look after her house and provide her with nutritious food. She was started on treatment for her osteoporosis, and her neighbours made sure that she had regular company.

*Alison – during the menopause*

Alison was only 54 when she found, to her amazement, that she had osteoporosis. A young grandma, she enjoyed babysitting for her daughter's two tearaway toddlers, aged four and two. She felt healthy, had kept herself fit with dancing classes, and prided herself on her figure which hadn't altered visually in 30 years. Her only health problem had been severe period trouble in her late thirties, which had led to a hysterectomy and an early menopause. She had taken that in her stride, in fact enjoying the freedom from a monthly cycle and the lack of any need for contraception. After a year of taking hormone replacement, she stopped it because she didn't feel the need for it. She was feeling well and had an active life, and didn't want to take hormones for the next 20 years or more.

It came as a complete surprise to her, therefore, that when she tripped over one of the four-year-old's toys in the playroom and stuck her hand out to break the fall, she broke her wrist. When she rose from the carpet, it was not so much the pain that she noticed but the 'dinner-fork' appearance of the back of her wrist. There was now a bend in it that had never been there before.

A quick visit to the local accident and emergency (A&E) unit showed that Alison had a 'Colles fracture' – the classical break in the wrist bones that comes from suddenly having to bear one's whole upper body weight on the wrist. The X-ray showed not only the break, but also the suspicion that the bones were very 'porotic' – they showed up much lighter on the X-ray than they should have at her age. The surgeons passed her back to her family doctor with the advice that she be investigated for osteoporosis, and left the decision on management to him.

Investigations (we will go into them later) showed that she had quite advanced osteoporosis, and she was put on several treatments and given advice on how she should live from then onwards so as to minimize the risks of any further fractures. That was four years ago. She is doing very well and there is evidence that her bones are strengthening as a result of her treatment. She is still looking after her grandchildren, though she says that soon they will be old enough to look after her. I know that feeling!

### Janine – the ballet dancer

Janine was a top-class ballet dancer, having danced leading roles in an internationally known company that travelled the world. At around five foot four, she was the perfect height for a ballerina, and she had kept her weight to a minimum throughout her career. I met her shortly after she retired from professional dancing and was teaching students. This still meant that she had to keep up her fitness level and her slim physique – not an easy combination to achieve, as it means keeping muscles strong without them bulking up in a masculine way. She managed it by strictly controlling what she ate. She had taught herself over the years not to respond to hunger by eating, and it showed. At 38 she was painfully thin.

Her main complaint was backache. Her back had begun to ache some months before seeing me, and she had put it down to 'wear and tear' – a favourite excuse for muscle and bone problems that is almost never correct. Using muscles and bones properly does not wear them out: on the contrary, it strengthens them and protects against their degeneration with age. Her immediate reason for the visit was that for the first time she was experiencing sciatica – pain down the back of her left leg.

She weighed just 44 kg (7 st). Asked to lie on the examination couch, she developed a severe pain when I raised her straight left leg (holding her at the ankle) when it reached a position only 30 degrees from the horizontal. Her ballet training had, of course, made her limbs very supple, but the muscles of the small of her back were stiff and tender on the slightest pressure.

I was worried about these findings, and because Janine was a professional dancer asked for an urgent appointment with our professor of orthopaedics at the university clinic. The diagnosis was a surprise to me, as I had believed until then that someone as active as a dancer would avoid osteoporosis because her bones would have become so strong. In fact, she had severe osteoporosis, and her back pain was caused by a crush collapse of the third and fourth vertebrae in her lower back. This had led to pressure on the nerves leading into the gap between these vertebrae – the main one of which is the sciatic. The pain was a direct result of her osteoporosis.

Janine eventually needed orthopaedic surgery to 'prop' up her vertebrae and was given medicines to replace the lost bone structure. She was also advised that her dancing days were over, for fear of other fractures in her spine. She admitted to us then that she had always had a struggle with her weight in her dancing years. She had been close to anorexic in her avoidance of food, and had often used cigarette-smoking as a way of curbing her appetite.

This combination of over-exercising, near-starvation and smoking was a powerful recipe for developing osteoporosis, and she was beginning to pay the penalty. She has now accepted that she must exercise less and eat well. She was given a target weight of 54 kg (8.5 st) and has been much happier and in much less pain since she achieved it. She still teaches dancing, and has added lessons on how to eat properly to her course. Today's ballet teachers are very much more aware than those of the last generation of how to protect their students' health.

*Gerry – a young man on steroids*

Gerry was 17 when he had his first attack of Crohn's disease. It was a sudden severe illness, during which he nearly died from loss of blood and fluids and a near-overwhelming infection. In intensive care for several weeks, he eventually pulled through, but at the expense of a series of operations and of times when the only food he could have was by intravenous drip. Crohn's disease is an acute inflammation of the bowel that leads to massive diarrhoea and bleeding, so that at one point he weighed less than 38 kg (6 st), despite his height of over six feet.

His recovery was long and drawn out, and he needed high doses of cortisone-like steroids to keep the bowel inflammation at bay. Slowly he became better and was allowed to leave hospital, but the steroids had to continue for at least a year, as he was having 'breakthrough' episodes of bloody diarrhoea. On his twentieth birthday he was well enough to have a party with his friends and, being a normal and active young man, he joined in the dancing. Halfway through a fairly vigorous dance, he felt a sudden pain in his back and had to sit down. The pain continued, and he knew enough about it (he had been warned by his doctors) to admit himself into the hospital unit, where the Crohn's specialist staff knew him well.

The pain was a fracture of a vertebra in the middle of his back. Gerry had advanced osteoporosis, a well-recognized side effect of long periods of high-dose steroid treatment. He had to spend some more weeks in hospital for the fracture to heal and was placed on intensive treatment to try to strengthen his bone structure. Sadly, he will not recover his lost height. Today, at 30, and free of Crohn's for the last five years, he is a full three inches shorter than he was at 17. He doesn't mind, as he is now living a completely normal life, and thinks that the loss of height is a small drawback of treatment that gave him back his life.

Gerry's case of osteoporosis caused by long-term treatment with steroids is not rare in people who need them for a chronic disease. It used to happen often in people who received oral steroids for asthma, in the days before inhaled steroids (which are given in doses hundreds of times lower than the tablets).

*Amanda – with thyroid trouble*

Amanda was always heavy, even as a schoolgirl, and she continued to put on weight as she had her children and entered her late thirties. Then she began to feel tired all the time, her hair started to fall out and her husband, Harry, noticed that the skin of her face had coarsened. It was a good indication of how low she had become mentally that she hadn't noticed the change herself.

Harry took her to the doctor (Amanda couldn't be bothered to go herself, and had to be cajoled into it). One look at Amanda was enough. Her doctor was shocked at the change in her face and her shape. She had gained 12.75 kg (28 lb) in the previous year, and looked dull and depressed.

The combination of weight gain, slowing physical and mental activities, and the coarsening of her features suggested one diagnosis to the doctor – failure of the thyroid gland to produce its hormone, thyroxine. The name for this is 'myxoedema', or hypothyroidism, and luckily it is easily treated. There is no need here to go into the causes of thyroid diseases: it is enough to say that the treatment is to give the missing hormone as a daily tablet. The response is usually dramatic, the patient feeling better and brighter in hours, and the facial and body shape changes beginning to reverse in a few weeks.

After a month, Amanda was a different woman. Harry had his wife back, and they were both delighted with the change. As a bonus, Amanda found that she was losing weight – and started to take a few extra thyroxine tablets each day to maintain her weight loss. For the first time in her life she felt slim, although she was still a big lady. She was enjoying herself, until she slipped while walking the dog. The dog, seeing a cat on a wall, ran for it. Unfortunately the lead wrapped itself around Amanda's legs, and she fell. By this time her reactions were fast enough for her to put her arm out to save herself, but she still hit the pavement with a thump, and shattered her forearm in doing so.

At the A&E department, the doctors were curious that a woman in her late thirties could have broken her arm so easily. When they heard her history of thyroid trouble, however, and she told them how much thyroxine she was taking, they quickly put two and two together. A bone scan showed quite advanced osteoporosis in her wrists, hips and spine.

Amanda learned from them that one side effect of overdosing yourself with thyroxine can be to reduce your bone strength. It is a relatively common problem for women who take the hormone principally to lose weight, rather than in the small dose that is needed to replace the lost hormone after thyroid failure. She was asked to see her doctor for a review of her medicine doses, and not to use the hormone as a slimming aid, as that might well increase her risk of a further fracture.

### Julie – with insulin-dependent diabetes

Julie has had Type 1 diabetes (childhood onset, or insulin-dependent diabetes) since she was eight years old. Her diabetes was well controlled in her early childhood, but as she reached her later teens it became much more difficult. She had to give herself several insulin injections a day, working out the dose on her blood glucose levels, which she measured herself using an insulin meter. Despite all her efforts, she was still having days when her glucose levels remained too high, and other days when she had 'hypo' attacks, so that she fainted from lack of glucose. She was a 'brittle' diabetic.

She remained brittle during her twenties and thirties, when she went through a 'stormy' pregnancy and at times was very ill. Julie and the baby survived; both she and her husband coped very well in the circumstances. The deterioration in her diabetes during the pregnancy left her with kidney damage, but she felt that her baby was worth it. The baby girl, Emma, is doing very well at school and appears to be none the worse for her experience in the womb.

However, Julie knows that one of the complications of poorly controlled diabetes is osteoporosis, and she is on long-term treatment to prevent it. She takes vitamin D and calcium supplements, eats well and exercises appropriately. So far her bone density measurements are only a little below average, and her diabetes team (her general practitioner and diabetes nurse, supported by the hospital consultant) are following them up. If they dip further, the team will consider a bisphosphonate drug treatment to prevent any future fractures. In the long-term future, she may need to be offered a pancreas/kidney transplant, but she is on other drugs to try to protect her kidney and postpone the surgery for as long as possible. Julie is realistic and accepts what the future will throw at her with courage. She has shown a lot of that in her first 40 years, and I don't doubt that she will continue to do so when the next crisis comes.

Osteoporosis is a relatively common complication of difficult-to-control Type 1 diabetes, and anyone with it should be aware of it. Wide awareness of this has made testing for bone density a routine in diabetes clinics.

Other illnesses that produce osteoporosis include an overactive parathyroid gland (hyperparathyroidism) and Cushing's syndrome.

The parathyroids (so called because they lie in the throat beside the thyroid) control the levels of calcium in the blood. When they are overactive, producing too much parathyroid hormone, calcium is leached out of the bones into the bloodstream and from there into other tissues, where it can form stones in the kidneys or deposit calcium layers in tissues such as muscle and blood vessel walls. People who present with osteoporosis outside old age are routinely tested for hyperparathyroidism, a blood test that will be described later in the chapter on diagnosis.

Cushing's syndrome, named after American physician Harvey Cushing, is a disorder of the adrenal glands. The adrenal glands make 'corticosteroids', a group of hormones that are collectively known to the public as cortisone or 'steroids'. There are two main types of cortisone: one, called glucocorticoids, helps to control the way the body uses glucose and fats, as energy or in storage; the second, mineralocorticoids, help control the way our bones use calcium. Too much mineralocorticoid activity leads to loss of bone structure – and osteoporosis. So when you are investigated for the cause of your osteoporosis, you will have your steroid levels measured to check on your adrenal gland function.

*John – the older man*
We mustn't forget the older man. Although the public perception of osteoporosis is that it is almost exclusively a disease of women, men get it too. However, because men's bones are stronger from the beginning, and because historically men had physically more strenuous jobs than women, the symptoms of the illness don't normally start until at least a decade later in life. The average woman with osteoporosis starts to have fractures in her seventies; for men the main burden of the disease starts in their eighties.

That doesn't mean they are too old for the illness to be worth treating. Although there are political pressures in the UK today on doctors to ration treatment in the elderly (so that scarce resources can be switched to younger people), treating osteoporosis in older men can bring great benefits in relief of pain and keeping them mobile.

That was the case for John, who tripped over a kerb while walking along his local main street, out shopping for his invalid wife, Helen. He picked himself up and struggled on, despite the severe pain in his leg and hip. A friendly shopkeeper was worried about him, and forced him to stay until an ambulance arrived. The diagnosis of a fractured shaft of femur was made at the hospital, and he was operated upon later that day. Within a few weeks he was back shopping, and fully functioning as Helen's carer. At 87 that isn't a bad achievement.

He is now taking daily vitamin D and calcium supplements and a bisphosphonate to keep his bone strength as high as possible, and he walks two or three miles three or four times a week. They are leisurely walks, with a stick, but they still help his bones and muscles, and he enjoys them.

John and Helen have accepted a lot more help in the house, with a friendly team of women from the local community helping with housework and meals, and keeping Helen company to give John a break once or twice a week. For the moment it's enough to state that they are both enjoying a better quality of life since John had his accident – and that is what matters.

So why should Jane, Alison, Janine, Gerry, Amanda, Julie and John, people of different ages with different lifestyles and backgrounds, all have developed osteoporosis? To understand the answer, we have to learn about the structure of bone and how it can be altered by our genetics and the way we live. This is explained in Chapter 2.

# 2

# Bones – their structure and how they can go wrong

## Blasts and clasts

Before we can understand osteoporosis, we need to know about bones. It's easy to misunderstand them. After all, when we excavate a grave or find a long-dead body all that is left are the bones – the skeleton. So it's a common mistake to believe that they are solid, permanent tissues that don't change much once we have become adults. People suppose that once we have grown to maturity, that's it for bones – they don't change much and form a solid basis for the rest of our tissues.

That's wrong. Bones, like every other tissue in our body, are constantly being broken down and renewed. We have a set of cells in our bones that build them up – producing new bone materials all the time. They are called 'osteoblasts'. And we have another, corresponding set of cells: the 'osteoclasts', which remove the old bone, disposing of their materials through the bloodstream. In children, who are growing, the osteoblasts are much more active than the osteoclasts, so that bone grows and strengthens throughout childhood into early adulthood.

The preponderance of bone-building over bone-reduction activity normally continues until early adult life, so that our bones are strongest and most dense in our early twenties. From then on it is usually downhill – the osteoclasts coming into their own gradually over the years. There is a slow decline in bone density (and therefore strength) from the thirties onwards, which continues at the same rate in men and women, except for the 'blip' during the menopause in women, when for a few years the decline is faster. As osteoporosis develops, the bone eventually becomes too weak to stand up to stresses such as falls and weight-bearing, and it breaks. Vertebrae, wrist bones and thigh bones take the brunt of the stresses, but osteoporosis is a generalized loss of bone strength, so all parts of the skeleton may be affected. We don't know this is happening, because bones don't have the sort of nervous system that could tell the brain that something is going wrong. That's why several of the people described in Chapter 1 were shocked to find that they were actually ill. They had had no symptoms until they had their first fracture.

Bone has two components. The outside of the bone is the cortex (Latin for the bark of a tree). It is the hardest and densest bony tissue, and provides the strength. Bones of men have a thicker cortex than those of women, and it is relatively thicker, too, in physically active than in sedentary people of either sex. The centre of the bone is the 'trabecular' bone, the structure of which, under the microscope, looks like a sponge. This central bone under normal conditions looks like a firm mesh of well-connected strands, with no visible breaks, gaps or holes. This is the area in which the osteoblasts and osteoclasts lay down new bone and 'resorb' (break down) old bone.

Figure 1 shows the structure of the bones most involved in osteoporosis – the neck of the femur (thigh bone) and the vertebrae. On the left in each case is normal bone, and on the right is bone affected by osteoporosis. Osteoporotic bone clearly has a thinner cortex and the trabecular bone is sparse, with broken strands of bone and many spaces. It doesn't take much imagination to see that the bone on the right is much more likely to snap under pressure than the one on the left.

Why does osteoporosis happen? Bone is constantly remodelling and repairing itself. As bone ages, it develops faults in its molecular structure. This is identified by osteoclasts, which

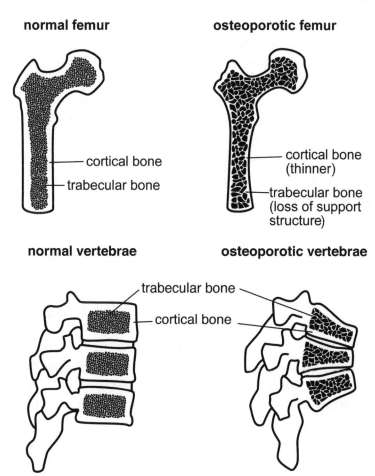

Figure 2.1 Bone structure, normal and osteoporotic

break the faulty area down by 'resorption', leaving a 'pit' behind – a hole in the bone. Osteoblasts then rush in and replace the lost bone with new material, replacing it and 'filling in' the pit bone. This process is exceptionally efficient for the first 40 years of our lives, but after this age the osteoblasts can't completely finish the job – there is a slight defect left in the bone. This doesn't matter much, because there is plenty of reserve strength in the remaining bone. What does matter is if our osteoblasts are even less efficient than they should be for our age. The pits become holes and larger defects. The spongy trabecular bone begins to look moth-eaten, and the cortex becomes much thinner.

This process of gradual failure of repair is a natural part of ageing. So why don't we all end up with osteoporosis? Much depends on the integrity of the various mechanisms that control the osteoblastic and osteoclastic processes. Knowing about them will help you to understand the treatments that you will be offered to reverse your bone loss.

## Calcium and vitamin D

Bones aren't only for keeping our bodies together, although without them we would just be big blobs of soft mushy tissue, like giant slugs. They have other functions, too. For example, we store in our bones around 98 per cent of our total content of calcium, the metal that is the main source of the hard material that makes up the bone. The marrow cavity in the trabecular bone is the site of manufacture of our red blood cells and most of our white blood cells, including the platelets that are vital to blood clotting and tissue repair.

To keep calcium levels in our bones that are adequate for maintaining their strength, we need vitamin D, the end effect of which is that it 'pushes' calcium from the bloodstream into the bone. A main source of vitamin D is sunlight – we make vitamin D when we expose our skin to light. A northern European needs just one hour of sunlight to make 400 units of vitamin D, an amount that lasts around two months in the body. If you are housebound, or are dark skinned and don't expose your skin to the sun in temperate climate zones, you will not create enough vitamin D in your skin to keep your bones healthy and strong – unless you eat enough vitamin D-containing foods every day. They are discussed in Chapter 8.

Here is where the explanation gets tricky. The vitamin D that is made in the skin or is eaten is 'inactive', in that it needs to be converted to other substances for it to do the job of placing more calcium into your bones. That conversion starts in the liver, which attaches a 'hydroxyl' (OH) molecule (a combination of a hydrogen and an oxygen atom) to it. It is now 25 hydroxy vitamin D (the 25 is the position in the molecule to which the OH molecule attaches). Even now, 25 hydroxy vitamin D (we will call it 25-HD for convenience) isn't active, and it is susceptible to degradation by various substances, such as certain drugs and many of the chemicals in tobacco.

It is only when calcium levels in the blood begin to drop that the body takes an active interest in the vitamin. The parathyroid glands (those ones I mentioned that lie beside the thyroid) detect the drop and secrete parathyroid hormone into the bloodstream. The kidneys pick up the parathyroid message, start to hold back on excreting calcium into the urine (so that calcium levels in the blood rise), and also act upon the circulating 25-IID as it passes through them. In the kidneys it becomes 1-alpha 25-dihydroxy vitamin D (1:25-DHD). It now has two OH molecules and has become the active vitamin at last.

To raise calcium levels in the body, 1:25-DHD acts in several ways. For example, when the bowel wall cells detect a higher amount of 1:25-DHD in the blood, they begin to extract more than their usual amount of calcium from the food that you have eaten. Blood calcium levels rise, and some of that calcium enters the bone.

This system is at its peak in children, who need the extra calcium to build their growing bones, but as we grow older the bowel's ability to absorb calcium becomes less efficient, and it does not react nearly as briskly to the message of the vitamin and the hormone. So after we reach maturity, we are less able to make good use of the calcium we eat.

We reach our peak bone mass (the time when our bones are strongest and most dense) at the age of 25.[1] After that, we start to lose bone mass. It is a precise age: it does not matter whether you are an athlete or a couch potato, male or female, that is the critical age. If you have not been absorbing enough calcium during your adolescence, you will not reach that peak mass of bone. That means that you enter your middle years with much lighter bones than you should have – and will reach the stage of osteoporosis earlier as your mechanisms for repair begin to fail. So poor eating habits, anorexia or slimming during adolescence and early adult life can start the process of osteoporosis and make it very difficult for you to avoid it later.

## Proteins

Calcium is not the only important component that helps you to achieve your peak bone strength. You need proteins, too, to make up the mass of tissue in the cortex and trabeculae within the bone. You will almost certainly consume them if you eat a good varied range of foods, but it is only too easy to forget the calcium component.

A normal portion, for example, of milk, cheese, ice cream or yogurt, contains about 250 to 280 milligrams (mg) of calcium. The recommended daily calcium intake for young children is 700 mg, or three dairy products. Adolescents and young adults up to the age of 25 need 1300 mg of calcium a day (six portions). Over that age the needs fall to 800 mg daily.

The need for calcium rises again in certain circumstances. Pregnant women need 1500 mg of calcium every day; breast-feeding women need 2000 mg. After the menopause, women need 1500 mg, as do all patients, men or women, who are recovering from a fracture.

It is difficult for younger people to accept that they must do something about their lifestyle *now* to prevent an illness that doesn't start to cause bother (unless they are very unlucky) until they are old. So when you tell a 13-year-old girl that she should eat and drink plenty of dairy products to prevent osteoporosis when she is 60, she will laugh at you. It is much more important to girls to be slim – and they link dairy foods to fatness. Nor is it any use trying to persuade them not to smoke, for exactly the same reason. The teenager who doesn't eat enough food containing enough calcium doesn't care that she will not achieve the bone mass she needs at 25. She has more exciting things to do than worry about her bones – after all, they feel perfectly sound to her, and 60 is a long way off.

## Phosphorus

The main mineral content of bone is not simply calcium, but calcium phosphate – a chemical combination of calcium and phosphorus. So an adequate intake of phosphorus is just as important to bone health as is that of calcium. Yet when was the last time you read in a woman's magazine about the need to eat or drink phosphorus-containing foods? I suspect this is the first time it has been brought to your attention.

We need enough phosphate in the bloodstream to build bone during our childhood and early adulthood. The units for measurement for minerals in our blood are millimoles per litre, or mmol/L, and a constant level of between 1.5 and 2.0 mmol/L of phosphate is needed to maintain the phosphate levels in bone. If blood phosphate levels drop below 1.5 mmol/L, then not enough of it is deposited in the bone, osteoblasts (bone-building cells) become less efficient, and osteoclasts, paradoxically, increase their rate of dissolving bone ('resorption'). So more bone is being resorbed than is being laid down – a powerful recipe for producing osteoporosis.

Phosphorus has an intimate relationship with calcium. The more phosphorus we eat in our food (for example in meat), the less calcium we excrete in our urine. Instead, we excrete any excess calcium through our faeces, thereby reducing our chances of developing a kidney stone, which is composed of calcium phosphate. We use phosphorus-containing supplements to treat people at high risk of kidney stones.

Phosphorus occurs in many foods, so it is an exception for our body level to be so low that it produces osteoporosis. The United States authorities recommend a daily intake of 700 mg. Very few people eat less than this on a regular basis, and most of them are elderly people who are not managing to feed themselves properly, perhaps because of failing mental health or extreme poverty. If they are eating too little food containing enough phosphorus, they are certainly eating too little calcium and good-quality protein as well, all of which are essential to bone health.

However, becoming low in phosphorus is not simply a matter of what you eat. Let's return to the relationship between calcium and phosphorus. Suppose you are diagnosed as having osteoporosis and are given a calcium supplement. Some calcium salts 'bind' phosphorus from our food in the gut, so that it cannot be absorbed into the body. The phosphorus remains in the gut, to be excreted in the faeces, and even though we are eating plenty of foods containing it, we can't use it to rebuild our bone. So the body takes phosphorus from muscles to replenish the bone. That doesn't matter too much in the elderly, but it may be one reason for people feeling weaker as they age.

Now add one of the new bone-building drugs, such as the bisphosphonates that stimulate osteoblasts and reduce osteoclast activity to the equation. As they build up bone material, they increase your need for extra phosphorus. If you are also taking calcium supplements, most of that calcium remains in the gut, where it binds closely to phosphorus, which prevents you from absorbing it. In 2002, R. P. Heaney and B. E. Nordin[2] calculated the amount of calcium supplement that would prevent all the phosphorus in our food from being absorbed.

It was only between 1 and 1.5 grams per day. At that level and above, the bowel becomes, in effect, an organ of phosphorus excretion – we start losing bodily phosphorus.

That sounds disastrous, but it is easily overcome. All you need to do is to drink an extra-large glass of milk a day, or to switch your calcium supplement to calcium phosphate. That provides the needed calcium and prevents further binding of phosphorus from food, so that some phosphorus becomes available to the bloodstream and bones. So if you are taking in extra calcium in the form of supplements, make sure you are taking the right type, as well as the correct amount. Frankly, it is better to eat foods containing plenty of calcium and phosphate rather than to depend on supplements for your main source of these two bone-building minerals.

## Female hormones

There is much more, however, to reaching that peak bone density than just eating calcium and phosphorus. Women's hormones play a huge part in preventing bone loss:[3] those who are still having periods lose only about 0.3 per cent of their skeleton each year. If they are taking normal amounts of calcium in their diet, there is no significant bone loss during these years. With the menopause comes a big change. The bone loss, without the support of hormones, rises dramatically to 2 per cent a year. This is a significant loss, amounting to over a quarter of the woman's bone mass in a mere 12 years if it continues.

Happily, in a normal menopause this period of massive bone loss does not last long. It continues for two or three years at most, then settles down to a less dramatic rate of around 1 per cent. However, women who have had their ovaries removed, for whatever reason, in their thirties and early forties, can lose bone at the highest rate for many years – perhaps 15 or more – if they do not have their missing hormones replaced.

The same applies to any woman who loses her periods early. Heavy smokers, for example, suffer a double whammy, in that the chemicals they inhale destroy much of their vitamin D before it becomes active, and at the same time can induce an early menopause. Smoking women tend to go through the menopause two to three years before non-smokers. Women such as professional athletes or gym and fitness fanatics who take part in such excessive physical activity that they lose their periods are in danger of bone loss despite using their bones to their maximum ability. Teenagers and young women with ano- rexia nervosa who starve themselves are not only eating far too little to keep up their bone mass, they also lose their hormonal protection. As they lose their periods (which is inevitable in anorexia), their bone loss accelerates to very high levels. They not only never reach their peak bone density at 25, they also have already started on the downward spiral of bone loss long before they are 20. It is really a desperate situation for them, apart from their other problems, psychological and physical.

I must add here a little about pregnancy and breast-feeding. It is true that during pregnancy women must deliver extra calcium from their diet to their developing baby. Babies in the womb are perfect parasites, taking all they need in nutrition from their mothers, who must eat healthily to provide enough calcium and protein for both of them. If they don't, their teeth can suffer. However, their extra hormones (oestrogen and proges- terone levels skyrocket during pregnancy) tend to protect them from developing osteoporosis during pregnancy. Breast-feeding mothers are obviously losing calcium in their milk and should eat healthily to replace it. As with pregnancy, it is unlikely that they will develop osteoporosis during that time, unless they are on extraordinarily faddy diets – and this will interfere, in any case, with their milk production.

## Teeth and jaws

The jaws, too, are a special case. If we lose our teeth early, we start to lose bone from our jaws. This is not true osteoporosis, but the result of the loss of the teeth from the sockets, leading to 'resorption' (loss) of bone caused by lack of use. 'If you don't use it, you lose it' is particularly true of bone. However, the most common reason for losing bone from our jaws is lifelong poor dental hygiene, with deposits of calculus (tartar) on the teeth below the gum line. This leads to chronic gum infection (gingivitis), with gradual loss of gum and bone. As the bone dies off, the roots of the teeth have less grip, and they begin to fall out.

We are probably the first generation to look after our teeth properly. Regular visits to our dentists, and in particular dental hygienists, have meant that many more of us are entering old age with most of our teeth intact. Those of us who do so should have no bother with receding jaws or with osteoporosis of the jaws.

## Exercise

Exercise is vital to bone health. Bones are sensitive to the load we put upon them. If we remain inactive for long periods, putting no load on our backs, hips and legs, we lose bone mass. The classic example of this is the astronaut, who is confined in a small space, weightless, for months on end. No matter how much exercise astronauts do in their capsule, when they return to earth they are exceptionally weak. Figures have been mentioned (although not confirmed in published medical texts, as far as I can find) of astronauts and cosmonauts losing as much as one-third of their bone mass in long periods in space.

Whether or not these reports are correct, it is true that inactivity – again the couch potato comes to mind – leads to weaker bones that are more than normally susceptible to fractures with minor falls and injuries.

However, it doesn't take much exercise to maintain our bones at a normal and healthy density. Even a daily walk, swim or cycle is enough. If you want to make them stronger, by all means push up your exercise levels to a faster walk, a climb, a jog or run, or dancing or any regular athletic exercise. Four or five days a week are enough – always have at least two days a week off to let your bones and muscles recover. The extra exercise will re-model your bones so that they can withstand the increased load on them – but only if you eat well, with plenty of calcium-containing food in your daily intake.

That applies at any age, even the very elderly. Studies in what the authors rather unkindly called 'aged women' have shown that they can actually increase their bone mass by regularly walking and dancing, and taking extra calcium as they do so.

## Stress and depression

There's no evidence that stress and depression contribute in a direct way to the cause of osteoporosis. People with them are no more likely to develop osteoporosis than those with a happy, contented lifestyle. However, the problems that osteoporosis can bring, with pain, loss of mobility and a poorer quality of life, can be a source of stress and depression. So doctors dealing with osteoporosis have to take into account the effect that it has on the mind, as well as the body. The best way to deal with that, of course, is to ease the symptoms, and how we do that is explained in a later chapter.

# 3

# Osteoporosis – the scale of the problem

In the United Kingdom every year, around 310,000 older people break a bone because they have osteoporosis. In the United States, the corresponding figure is 1.5 million, of which 700,000 are vertebral, 300,000 are in the hip and 200,000 in the wrist. In Switzerland, osteoporosis-related disability causes more inactive days in bed than strokes, heart attacks, breast cancer or obstructive lung disease.[1]

These are mind-blowing figures, but they are not easy to relate to one's own chances of having a fracture. So it is probably better to explain the burden of illness caused by osteoporosis in a different way – by calculating each person's risk of a fracture in his or her lifetime. Of these, hip fractures cause the most distress and lead to the most deaths, the longest periods of disability and the highest risk of permanent dependence on others. Spinal fractures (mostly collapsed vertebrae) are less common, but cause considerable disability. The average age at which women experience their first fracture is 81, when they can expect, on life expectancy figures, to live another 8.7 years. For women the lifetime risk of dying from a hip fracture is the same as that of dying from breast cancer, and men over 50 are at greater risk of osteoporosis-induced fracture than they are of prostate cancer. The World Health Organization has identified osteoporosis as second only to cardiovascular disease as a leading health-care problem.

So there is every good reason to try to prevent such fractures and to treat them, in order to give men and women a good chance of returning to their normal lifestyle.

The UK isn't unique in its low-key approach to osteoporosis. Osteoporosis affects 200 million people worldwide, and in almost every country it is under-recognized and under-treated, mainly because it is a 'silent' disease until it causes its first fracture. This is a life-changing event for so many people, who never again feel that they can walk down a street safely and are much more insecure than before when they attempt normal everyday activities. If you can prevent yourself from breaking a bone, you can extend your normal active quality of life for many years.

By 2025 a quarter of Europe's population will be over 65 years old;[2] the extent of the problem we face in the years to come can only be imagined. Today, 40 per cent of women can expect one day to suffer a fracture of the wrist, hip or spine. By the time they are 80, one in five women will already have had a hip fracture, a figure that rises to half by the age of 90. Women older than 85 are eight times more likely than women aged 65 to 74 years to be admitted to hospital because of a hip fracture. A 70-year-old woman is five times more likely than a younger woman to fracture her hip. That's mainly because she is less steady on her feet than a younger woman, and therefore will fall more often. Most hip fractures are the result of a fall, although, as I explained in the introduction, some people spontaneously break their hips while walking, and then fall.

Although most fractures in people with osteoporosis are of the hip, wrist and vertebrae, a substantial minority of them are in other bones. They depend to a great extent on how the person falls. An awkward trip at the kerb when crossing the road, or over a loose carpet in the home, or over a pet cat or dog, can snap the shaft of the thigh bone (the femur), the ankle or the middle of the lower leg (tibia and fibula). Putting your hand out to save a fall can snap the collar bone (clavicle) or the middle of the humerus (the upper-arm bone). Any break in a bone after

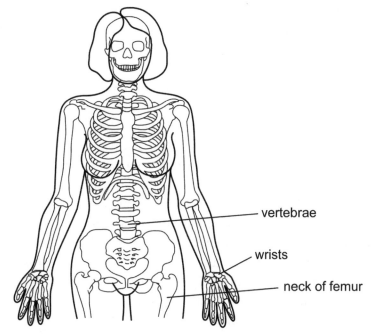

vertebrae

wrists

neck of femur

**Figure 3.1 Sites of main fractures in osteoporosis**

a fall in an older person raises the suspicion of osteoporosis, as bones even in older people should normally be strong enough to withstand such an impact.

As the population ages, therefore, we are going to see a huge increase in the numbers needing treatment – unless we take strong action to reverse these risks. As doctors, it is part of our task to spot the potential osteoporosis patient in our daily surgeries, and to take action before the calamity occurs. How we recognize her (and occasionally, him) is described in the next chapter. It will give you an insight into whether you are at high risk.

The next few chapters describe ways in which we are trying to reduce the risks of fracture due to osteoporosis in our patients. But it is a team effort, and you, the potential patients, need to play your part in it. You can help yourselves by following the right eating habits and exercising in the right way. We can help you by diagnosing osteoporosis before you break a limb or vertebra, and by giving you treatments that will strengthen your bones and prevent a break.

Sadly, today, we fail to diagnose most people with osteoporosis early enough, and even when we do make the diagnosis (usually after a fracture) we do not give them the full and correct treatment. Treating a fracture is not just a matter of putting the bones back together again (there are several ways of doing this, from inserting nails and screws to replacing the parts of the bones that are broken with artificial materials, such as replacing a joint). If we don't also then face up to the cause of the fracture – the process that is making the bones too porous – the person will have more fractures. Everyone who has a broken bone as they grow older needs full investigation into why it has happened, and then intensive treatment to try to ensure that it doesn't happen again. That treatment includes supervision of eating habits, an exercise programme to get the person fit again, and drugs to strengthen the bones – which will be described in detail in Chapter 11.

How poorly we doctors have been implementing such tests and treatments has been shown by two large studies. In the first, K. B. Freeman and his colleagues[3] reported that of 1,162 women who had broken their wrists, only 24 per cent had had a diagnostic evaluation or treatment of the fracture. Only 2.8 per cent had a scan to measure their bone density and only 22.9 per cent were eventually given anti-osteoporotic drugs.

In the second, G. M. Kiebzak and colleagues, in an article entitled 'Undertreatment of osteoporosis in men with hip fractures'[4] showed that although women were treated inadequately for osteoporosis, men were neglected to an even greater degree. Only 27 per cent of the men in their study of 363 people with hip fractures were given anti-osteoporotic treatment after their fractures, compared with 71 per cent of the women.

There is obviously a sore need for us to do better. We need to identify the people most at risk before they have their fracture, and in the next chapter I describe how doctors approach this task on both sides of the Atlantic.

# 4

# Risk assessment and change

So how close to a calamitous bone fracture are you? By the end of this chapter you will have a good idea.

General practitioners in the United Kingdom are now very well aware that preventing fractures in older people is a priority. Naturally, much of that awareness comes from their experience of the difficulties their patients encounter after breaking a bone, and the need to avoid fractures if at all possible. But we also have experts in the field to guide us on how to do so, and we are fortunate in the UK to have Anthony D. Woolf, Professor of Rheumatology at the Peninsula Medical School, the Royal Cornwall Hospital, Truro, as one of them.

In their *British Medical Journal* article,[1] Professor Woolf and his colleague, Professor Kristina Akesson of Malmo University Hospital, Sweden, laid down a set of rules for general practitioners. These rules covered when and how to assess the risk of future fracture from osteoporosis in elderly people. I have set them out here, only slightly changed to make them more suitable for a non-medical audience.

*Question 1:* Are you concerned about this person's risk of fracture?

If the answer is no, then simply give lifestyle advice.

If it is yes, then three questions must follow. They are:

*Question 2:* Is the person at risk of falling? This is assessed from whether or not the person:

(a) has fallen within the last year;

(b) has weak legs;

(c) has a poor gait (walks awkwardly and tentatively);

(d) has impaired balance;
(e) has limbs that are not well co-ordinated;
(f) has poor eyesight.

*Question 3:* Has he or she had a fracture of the wrist, upper arm or vertebra after a minor accident, or associated with known osteoporosis?

*Question 4:* Is he or she at risk of osteoporosis? This is assessed from:
(a) a low body mass index (underweight for his or her height);
(b) long-term treatment with cortisone-like steroid drugs;
(c) reduced lifetime exposure to oestrogens, such as a menopause before the age of 45;
(d) long-term loss of periods, failure to develop during teenage years;
(e) a history in the mother's family of hip fracture;
(f) other illnesses linked to osteoporosis such as: rheumatoid arthritis; bowel malabsorption disorders such as coeliac disease, Crohn's disease, previous bowel surgery; or long-term immobilization (as in any chronic illness forcing the person to rest).

If the answer is yes to any of questions 2, 3 and 4, then your doctor must take several actions. The first is to take some time exploring your lifestyle:

• Do you have healthy eating habits?
• Are you active physically and socially?
• Do you eat enough foods containing calcium?
• Do you expose yourself enough to the sun?
• Do you do any weight-bearing exercise, such as walking briskly, running, even doing weight training?

If your answers show that you do none of the above, then you must change. You are heading for a fall, and a fracture.

In addition, your doctor will ask about smoking and drinking. If you smoke, then you must stop – it is no use cutting down, that doesn't work. I've devoted a chapter to smoking for the tobacco users, because stopping smoking is a crucial step in preventing fractures. If you don't stop, you are inviting trouble.

You may also be asked about cannabis. Have you ever smoked cannabis, and if so, for how long and how much? This is relevant to your bone health today, even perhaps 30 or 40 years later. Professor Stuart Ralston and his research team at Aberdeen University (he is now at Edinburgh) found that smoking cannabis will promote osteoporosis.[2] They showed that, as well as curbing appetite, chemicals in cannabis (cannabinoids) stimulate resorption of bone. Giving mice chemicals that mimic cannabis-smoking led to loss of bone mineral density. More important, blocking the receptors for cannabinoids in the mice prevented this bone loss, a fact that Professor Ralston hopes will lead to effective treatments for human osteoporosis. He is now hoping to find evidence of developing osteoporosis among long-term cannabis users.

As for drinking, a small amount of alcohol – no more than one or two small glasses of wine a day with meals – should be your limit. If you are unsteady on your feet and have some balance problems, then you should cut out alcohol altogether, as even small amounts of it will heighten your unsteadiness and make it much more likely that you will fall.

The next step in the assessment is to determine whether you can take long-term treatment to reduce your risk of fracture.

If you are too old and frail to do so, then your doctor will still prescribe calcium and vitamin D pills to be taken daily, and will also help you with exercises to train your balance and co-ordination. This will usually be supervised by a specialist nurse or a physiotherapist.

If you are willing and able to take long-term treatment, then you will be asked to have a bone density measurement, the result of which will determine your specific treatment recommendations. Needless to say, the calcium and vitamin D treatment and balance training will apply to you, too.

It can't be emphasized too strongly that simply prescribing drugs to strengthen bones is only a small part of the battle against the fractures caused by osteoporosis. You must also alter your lifestyle, and often your closest environment (your home), so that you minimize all chances of falling. It isn't easy, but it can be done, and the next few chapters will explain how to do it.

## Problems provoking falls

It is worthwhile here going more deeply into the risks of falling. Old age, sadly, rarely produces just one health problem. As we age, several of our bodily systems don't work as well or as smoothly as they used to. So your doctor will be examining you for what we call 'intrinsic' factors that can increase your risk of falling and breaking a bone.

They include poor control of posture because our nervous system doesn't always know exactly where it is 'in space'. We get up and sit down more slowly because we don't quite know where our body parts are in relationship to the furniture. We shake as we do so, because our muscles aren't working in complete co-ordination. Our reaction time to what is happening around us is slower, our legs are weaker, and we may have arthritis or stiffness that makes walking quickly and efficiently just a bit more difficult than it used to be. One test doctors do measures co-ordination, balance, position sense and reaction times in one easy action. You will be asked to stand up from a chair without using your arms, walk several paces, return and sit down again. This is the 'get up and go' test. If you show no unsteadiness or difficulty performing it, then your nervous system is still intact, and there's no worry that you are especially prone to falling.

Along with problems in our limbs, we may also be developing eyesight problems. Cataracts are common causes of blurred vision in the over-seventies, as is macular degeneration (a form of gradual onset of blindness in which we lose our central vision, and can only see around the periphery of what we used to see). It is so easy, then, to trip over a rug or a chair that we couldn't see sharply enough.

To make matters even worse, the seventies are the age of 'transient ischaemic attacks' (TIAs) in which tiny clots of blood pass through the arteries of our brain, leading to very short periods of unconsciousness. We fall, often without warning, waking up on the floor with no memory of what happened. If our bones are brittle because of osteoporosis, a TIA can often lead to a fracture.

Some treatments for high blood pressure, yet another common ailment as we grow older, can give 'postural hypotension' – a 'faint' that hits us as we stand up from a sitting or lying position, often as we get out of a bath. It is the result of the blood pooling in the abdomen and failing to reach the brain, which responds by shutting down for a short while, hence the faint. Postural hypotension falls, like TIAs, are also relatively common causes of fractures.

Heart arrhythmias – brief periods when the heart is beating in an abnormal rhythm – can also lead to sudden loss of blood flow to the brain, and a fall that might produce a fracture. They, too, like TIAs and postural hypotension, are more common as we age.

So it should go without saying that when someone falls for the first time and has broken a bone, or even if he or she has just been badly shaken, it is incumbent on the doctor to find the cause of the fall. Osteoporosis may be the reason for the bone breaking, but it is essential to find out why the person has fallen in the first place. Could it have been a TIA, or a reaction to a blood pressure-lowering drug, or a heart arrhythmia? That first fall is only the start of a necessary series of investigations to find the cause, and when it is found, to try to correct it and prevent other falls. The answer may be something as simple as a small dose of aspirin a day to prevent the clotting that provokes a TIA, or a change in the blood pressure medication, or the prescription of a drug to correct the arrhythmia.

## Getting your home right

Most falls happen in your home. If you are unsteady, and have poor eyesight, it's easy to trip over something left on the floor. Every family doctor will sigh at the memory of being called to a patient, often a friend of many years, who has tripped over a grandchild's toy, or the edge of a loose rug, a pet, a cord for a telephone or an electrical appliance, like a heater or a lamp. Slippery kitchen or bathroom floors are another hazard in the home, as are loose stair carpets. Bad lighting, stairs that are too steep and bedroom furniture that is in the way when you want to get quickly to the bathroom in the night are all too familiar fracture-awaiting obstacles in the home.

This, too, is part of the assessment your doctor will want to make in assessing your risk of a fracture. You may be asked to allow the local nurse to assess your home and advise you on how to make it safer. It is difficult to know how many broken bones such changes have prevented, but it must run into hundreds of thousands.

Of course, outdoors is just as full of hazards as the average home. Uneven pavements, poor street lighting, icy conditions, difficulties getting on and off public transport or into and out of private cars, are all regular sources of falls. Just a little extra care when you know you are at risk can make a lot of difference.

## If you have had a fall (or two)

If you are getting on in years and have had a fall, or fear that you might fall because you have become unsteady, your doctor must be told.

You will then be subjected to a 'fall evaluation', the form of which has been standardized (as so much in modern medical practice is nowadays), but which is adapted to each individual's needs. You will be asked about the circumstances that led to the fall – did you trip over an obstacle, or was it a sudden, unexpected incident out of the blue? Have you recently started on new medicines, perhaps for your heart or circulation or blood pressure? Do you have any problem with your joints or muscles that makes you unsteady on your feet, or gives you difficulty in walking or lifting your feet high enough to go up stairs or step over things easily?

Having answered these questions, you will be fully examined. The examination will take in assessments of your nervous system and muscles and joints and how well they are co-ordinated. Your doctor will then know a lot about your balance and your muscle strengths and weaknesses, and whether your nerves of sensation (particularly those which tell your brain where your feet and the rest of your body are in relation to the space around you) are working normally.

Your mental state will also be assessed. This includes your mood (are you depressed or anxious?) and your intellectual capacity (are you less able mentally than you were?).

Your heart and circulation will be examined. How steady, or regular, is your heartbeat? Is there any abnormality of rhythm? Is your blood pressure within the normal range? It should not be too high, which is very common, but it should also not be too low. This is much less common, but is a source of fainting and therefore of falls. Your doctor may even massage a spot in your neck called the carotid sinus, to see if your pressure changes. If it does, you may have postural hypotension. This causes you to fall when you move suddenly from the horizontal to the vertical, because your blood pressure falls when you do, and this sharply reduces the blood flow to your brain.

If the results of any of these tests do indicate that you are at risk of further falls, and that osteoporosis might be an underlying cause, then you will be asked to have a bone density scan, and perhaps other tests as well. These are described in the next chapter.

# 5

# Making the diagnosis

## Bone mineral density (BMD)

There is just one absolute way to make the diagnosis of osteoporosis – to measure your bone mineral density, or BMD. The
underlying cause of osteoporosis is loss of the minerals that
make bones strong: when that happens the bones become full of
holes, or pores, and become less dense. Look on the osteoporotic
bone in cross-section like a ciabatta loaf, rather than a whole-
meal one, and you get the idea.

How do we measure bone density? That's the problem. In
straight uncomplicated X-rays of your bones, they may appear
lighter than normal on the film, but there are too many vari-
ables in this sort of assessment (including minor variations, for
example, in the film, or overlying muscle shadows) to come to
any definite conclusion from them. However, a straight X-ray
can certainly point to the diagnosis with a fair degree of prob-
ability. It can show, for example, a vertebra that has collapsed
in on itself in a person with back pain in whom a fracture
hasn't been suspected as its cause. (Most back pain is muscular,
rather than bony, in origin.) It can also show to the trained eye
a strong suggestion of under-mineralization in a wrist or thigh
bone, but neither is definitive, and it does not give a measure of
the loss of bone or of the risk of future fracture – which is often
the main purpose of the investigation.

# DXA (or DEXA)

To obtain such a measure we need 'single and dual X-ray absorptiometry', or DXA for short. Doctors commonly call it DEXA. This isn't the book to explain how different it is from normal X-rays: it is enough to state that it is accepted worldwide as the most accurate measure of BMD. If you are technically minded, then you can read the paper that established DXA as the method of choice for measuring bone density, or 'densitometry'.[1]

DXA is used to measure 'whole body' BMD and BMD at the hip, and can be used to predict the risk of future fractures with considerable accuracy. However, the result is given in an unusual way, unlike those of other tests that simply give a figure above or below which the result is abnormal.

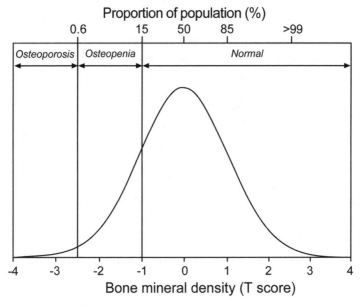

**Figure 5.1 Bone mineral density**
Source: The Lancet, 1 June 2002, p. 1930.

This is because a 'normal' BMD varies widely among individuals. The range of BMD measurements in a population of a particular age is wide. They follow a 'bell-shaped curve' in which most readings fall within the upper part of the bell shape, but a few are dotted around the 'rim' of the bell (see Figure 3).

If your BMD falls within the 95 per cent of readings that make up the 'body' of the bell, it is assumed to be normal. However, if it is down near the 'rim', to the left of the main part of the curve by what mathematicians call minus one standard deviation (–1SD), then you have a low bone mass – not yet osteoporosis, but a condition called 'osteopenia'.

If you are further outside the main curve, at a point beyond two and a half standard deviations to the left (–2.5SD), then you have osteoporosis.

The measurement is called the 'T score', in deference to the science of statistics, which defined and labelled the properties of bell-shaped curves that arise from the analysis of populations.

The World Health Organization (WHO) and the International Osteoporosis Foundation (its address is on p. 104) came together to create four diagnostic categories for women undergoing DXA measurement. They are:

- Normal: a BMD at the hip less than 1SD below the mean for normal young adult females (T score above –1).
- Low bone mass (osteopenia): a hip BMD more than 1SD but less than 2.5SD below the young adult female mean (T score below –1 but above –2.5).
- Osteoporosis: a hip BMD score more than 2.5SD below the young adult female mean (T score below –2.5).
- Severe osteoporosis: hip BMD 2.5SD or more below the young adult female mean plus one or more fragility fractures (T score below –2.5).

As explained previously, women lose bone mineral faster after the menopause than in their young adult lives. Yet 15 per cent of the young healthy female population in the developed world are already in the low bone mass group with T scores of between –1 and –2.5.[2] One in 200 already has severe osteoporosis. However, the T score taken at one site in the body only reflects the risk of fracture at that site. So a T score of –2.5 at the hip may not be matched by the same score in a vertebra, mainly because we are biological beings (thankfully) and grow differently in different sites of our bodies. Doctors therefore choose the site we think most likely to be the cause of a fracture when asking for a DXA test. If the patient's predominant symptom is back pain, then a vertebral DXA is taken. If we are more concerned about the hip, then the hip bones are the sites for the test.

For most people the hip DXA is the gold standard for making the diagnosis as it has the highest predictive value for future hip fracture, and is the most severe complication of osteoporosis. DXA at other sites is usually requested in people with known osteoporosis and for whom there is a special reason (such as pain in the area) for wishing to assess fracture risk there.

Although these decisions about the use of DXA for the diagnosis of osteoporosis have followed extensive studies in women, they are also relevant to men. Some studies have suggested that the curve for BMD differs between the sexes, so that one has to use different criteria in men to calculate their risk of fracture. However, it seems from the few studies available in men that the risk of hip fracture is similar for men and women for any given BMD. We therefore use the same cut-off point, a T score of –2.5, in men as in women.

## Bone ultrasound

DXA is not the only way to measure bone density. Ultrasound (the use of sound waves rather than X-rays) can be used to measure bone density. It is most widely used to measure the density of bone at the heel by measuring the speed of the ultrasound waves through it. This technique avoids the use of X-rays, but it can't be used to diagnose osteoporosis. It is a support, however, to the overall tests that give doctors an idea of fracture risk in older women.

## CT scan

Everyone has heard of 'CAT' scans. The letters mean 'computer-assisted tomography'. It is more often abbreviated by doctors to 'CT' scan, standing for 'computed tomography', and it is now adapted to give a quantitative measure of osteoporosis, particularly of the spine. The basic difference between CT scans and DXA is that the former gives a 'volumetric' density, whereas the latter gives an 'area-adjusted' result. In simpler terms, this means that CT is in 3-D, while DXA is a two-dimensional test, of an area of bone rather than a volume. CT also gives a more detailed image of the internal 'cancellous' bone than DXA (see Chapter 2 on normal and osteoporotic bone structure). As cancellous bone is much faster to respond to treatment than the outer cortex, CT scans are more often used to monitor the results of treatment than to make the initial diagnosis. They are also able to distinguish osteoporosis from degenerative bone disease more easily than does DXA, which is a drawback for DXA when the spine is being examined.

However, CT has major drawbacks, such as a higher exposure of the patient to radiation, difficulties with controlling the quality of the pictures, and very much higher cost than DXA. Cost does come into the decision to use it, as it would be impossible for any health system to afford CT scans for all the many thousands of people needing investigation for probable osteoporosis.

## Using the results to predict your risk

What really matters in osteoporosis is not the fact that you have the bone problem, but whether or not it will cause you pain and distress – in effect, will it cause you to break a bone? Measuring the bone density is therefore only useful in so far as it helps to establish your risk and to direct your doctor towards the most effective treatment. Your BMD result is not taken in isolation, but is looked at along with other test results that will add further information about your likelihood of a fracture.

The fact that the diagnosis is made from a cut-off figure such as a T score of –2.5 on DXA isn't completely satisfactory. If you have a score that is better than this (say –2.0), it doesn't mean that you have no chance of having a fracture, and there are people with scores of –2.8 who never fall or break a bone. So the T score is an arbitrary guide, not an absolute that something will go wrong if it goes beyond –2.5. However, it is true that the further your score drops below –2.5, the higher your risk of fracture. Your risk of fracture rises between 1.5- and three-fold with each SD decrease in BMD. This means that at the higher rate (it depends on age) a person with a T score of –3 has three times the risk of a fracture compared to a person with a T score of –2. A T score of –4 carries a nine-fold rise in risk over the score of –2.

It isn't unusual in medicine to calculate risk in this way. For years we have known that for each percentage point rise in blood pressure the risk of stroke from a bleeding blood vessel in the brain rises two percentage points. So a very high blood pressure indicates a very high stroke risk. Yet there are some people who have a constantly high blood pressure who never have a stroke until extreme old age. The problem is that it is impossible to determine beforehand who will be the survivors and who will not, so it is standard practice, and very sensible, to treat every person with high blood pressure as if he or she is one of the potential victims.

The same logic applies to the person with osteoporosis. If your DXA scan shows a T score of –2.5, you need seriously to consider preventive treatment, even if you have not yet had a fall or a fracture. However, you still need other tests to help confirm your risk, and to see if there are any underlying causes other than primary osteoporosis that are making your bones lose their mineral content.

## Urine tests for osteoporosis

We now have urine tests that will check on how much bone you are building up (bone formation) and how much you are resorbing (breaking down) – markers of osteoblast and osteoclast function. They are called collectively 'bone turnover markers'.

The bone formation markers are: total alkaline phosphatase, bone isoenzyme alkaline phosphatase, osteocalcin, and procollagen propeptides of type I collagen. Don't be put off by their names. They are all normal substances that are involved in the formation of bone, and in people who are keeping a good balance of bone building and bone resorption their levels in the urine keep within well-defined limits. The urinary markers of bone resorption are hydroxyproline, pyridinium crosslinks and their associated peptides. The higher their levels in your urine, the faster you are losing bone mineral, and therefore the greater your risk of a fracture.

If your doctor is concerned with your bone turnover, he or she will request the local biochemistry department to measure these, or at least some of these, markers in your urine. Taken along with your BMD, the results of your tests will help to predict your risk of fracture. If you have a low BMD and your urinary markers are outside the normal range for the laboratory, your risk could double or more, depending on the extent of the rise.

## Risks linked to other illnesses

Once the suspicion of osteoporosis has been raised, your doctor then has to seek a cause for the excessive loss of bone. If you are a relatively young man or woman, you will have your blood tested for your levels of sex hormones – oestrogens in women and testosterone in men. If they are low, this could be a pointer to your bone loss.

Low hormone levels in women are linked to a premature menopause, or to previous surgery on the ovaries, chemotherapy or radiotherapy. In men, low testosterone levels are found in inherited conditions such as Klinefelter's syndrome, in which the testes do not develop correctly and do not produce any significant testosterone. Low pituitary gland function ('hypopituitarism') and a high output of prolactin (a hormone secreted by the pituitary, and used to produce breast milk in women – what it does for men is unclear) may predispose to osteoporosis in men. Probably the commonest cause of osteoporosis in men today, however, is the anti-testosterone treatment given for prostate cancer. Although it is very successful in keeping some prostate cancers under control, it has the side effect of inducing excess bone mineral loss. So if you are on hormone treatment for prostate cancer, you should have a risk assessment for osteoporosis, usually using DXA.

In both sexes, prolonged treatment with steroid hormones is a cause of osteoporosis. The loss is fastest and greatest in the first few months of treatment, and particularly affects the vertebrae. When steroid tablets taken by mouth were given routinely for asthma, many people with asthma became osteoporotic, and the price they paid for their asthma relief was often crush fractures of the vertebrae, with shortening of the spine and loss of several inches in height. The change from pills to inhalers, in which the dose is hundreds of times lower and most of it remains within the lungs, has caused this form of osteoporosis almost to disappear in people with asthma.

However, it remains a risk for people who still must take steroids by mouth, such as some transplant recipients, people with long-term kidney disease, and people with blood disorders or immune problems. If the dose of prednisolone, the commonest form of steroid, is kept below 7.5 mg per day, the risk of vertebral fracture is minimized.

Overactivity of the thyroid gland is also associated with osteoporosis, so your doctor will probably check on that, too, with blood tests. In the past, a common cause of osteoporosis was partial gastrectomy – the operation to remove most of the stomach that was almost universal for stomach ulcers before we learned how to treat them successfully medically. Without two-thirds of their stomachs, patients were unable to digest enough calcium, phosphorus and proteins to keep their bones healthy. Some older men and women who had such stomach surgery in the 1950s and 1960s may be gradually slipping into osteoporosis without knowing it – until they have their first fracture. If you have had such surgery, please get a check-up.

Other illnesses not directly linked to osteoporosis but that make people prone to falling include arthritis, partial paralysis due to a stroke, Parkinson's disease, vertigo (dizziness), alcoholism, blindness and dementia. If you have an illness like this that may cause you to fall and have osteoporosis as well, you need special attention and treatment to try to keep your bones strong so that when you do fall, they won't break. Trials have shown that even when elderly women fall in the home, if they have a normal bone density they have only a 1 per cent chance of a fracture. If they are in the severe category of osteoporosis, that risk rises by ten-fold or even more, so it is important to identify any condition that you might have that could cause you to fall.

Once the diagnosis has been established, how should you be treated? Much depends on your age, your risk of a bone fracture over the next ten years, and for how long you wish to be treated with powerful drugs aimed at driving mineral back into your bone. No drug is without side effects, and your osteoporosis would have to be severe, and you would have to be at high risk (say at least a 10 per cent risk of fracture each year), before you would wish to be on one of the bone-strengthening drugs for the rest of your life. This is especially so if you are still relatively young.

Before describing these treatments in detail, therefore, the next chapters will deal with the consequences of osteoporotic fractures, and what you can do for yourself, in eating habits, exercise and lifestyle changes, to reduce your chances of developing them.

# 6

# The problems with fractures

The over-riding aim when you have osteoporosis is to avoid broken bones, especially the hip, the wrist and the vertebrae. That's not just because the fractures themselves are painful: they can also have consequences that make you feel that you will never be quite the same again.

## Hips

Take a hip fracture first. It happens, on average, to people around the age of 80. At that age, you tend to lean slightly backwards or sideways when you walk, which makes you more likely to fall on one hip. As the fall obviously takes you by surprise, and your reactions are naturally slower than they used to be, you don't have time to put out your hands to break the fall, and the hip is the first part of you to hit the ground. The impact snaps it.

There is another scenario, less common but just as painful. As I mentioned earlier, in some cases the hip snaps first because it has become so brittle that it can no longer bear your weight as you walk.

However it happens, a broken hip is nearly always very painful and needs hospital admission. Today it is always operated on. If the two broken ends of the bone are still roughly in line, the break can be bridged with a metal plate fixed with pins, so that you keep the 'head' of your thigh bone (the femur) and the socket into which it fits in the pelvis. If the two broken surfaces are not in line, it is often easier for the patient and for healing to replace the femoral head with an artificial one.

44

Because you are likely to be frail by the time you have your operation, you will probably spend about three weeks in hospital recuperating, and several months slowly recovering your previous health. The figures are stark. Around one in five people who have a first hip fracture die within the next six months. Of the survivors, only a quarter recover enough to get back to their old lifestyle. One-third lose their independence permanently, most needing nursing-home care. The others need assistance at home to do many of their ordinary everyday tasks.

## Wrists

On average, broken wrists affect people in the decade before they break their hips. They are still fast enough to break a fall with their hands – hence the break, as the wrist bone can't take the sudden jolt. Most wrist fractures recover well, but the period just after the break can be difficult. Sometimes the broken ends don't heal in perfect alignment, leaving the wrist looking deformed, although it probably works reasonably efficiently.

Broken wrists are usually 'fixed' with a rigid splint, such as plaster of Paris or a more modern equivalent. One in three women with a broken wrist develop 'algodystrophy' afterwards, with pain, tenderness, swelling and stiffness in the hand. This can last for several years and is very difficult to treat. Affected women feel they can't use the hand as they used to. Knitting, crochet and similar skills become impossible for them – a big disadvantage if these were a particular interest.

## Vertebrae

Osteoporotic vertebral fractures differ from those in the hip and wrist because they take the form of a gradual collapse of the bone in the spinal column. The 'bodies' of normal vertebrae are cylinders with vertical sides and horizontal upper and lower surfaces. When they become osteoporotic, the central area of cancellous bone disintegrates as it fails to bear the weight of the body above it. The perfect cylindrical shape becomes distorted, to become wedge-shaped or with a 'dip' in the middle. The overall effect is for the affected vertebra to be thinner, losing its height, and making the person shorter and often bent forward.

The symptoms caused by vertebral osteoporosis vary. Some people feel no pain, but do notice that they are becoming shorter and more bowed with age. Others are in severe pain, often continuous. Yet others have intermittent pain of varying intensity. We don't know why the same apparent change can have such different outcomes: it is not simply the result of pressure on a nerve.

When it does occur, the pain spreads from the back, at the level of the vertebra affected, around the body to the front at the same level or just below it. It is at its most severe for some weeks, then usually dies away over months, or in extreme cases, years. If you are very unfortunate, you may have permanent discomfort.

As back pain is very common, and vertebral collapse due to osteoporosis is often painless, if you have severe back pain and an osteoporotic vertebral collapse the two may not be connected. The pain is just as likely to come from a disc problem or arthritis, or even from other more distant problems (such as prostate or kidney disease) as from the osteoporosis. So don't be surprised if your doctor wants to investigate your back pain further, despite your obvious osteoporosis. For example, spine fractures due to osteoporosis do not cause sciatica (in which the pain is in the back of the leg). Most sciatica is caused by muscle spasms in the back or by swollen discs (the discs of cartilage that act as shock absorbers between the vertebrae).

For most women, and for men too, the most distressing symptom of vertebral osteoporosis is the loss of height. As several vertebrae become affected, this loss can be as much as six inches – women can go from tall to short in a few years. Along with the shortening comes a 'hump' on the back as the spine curves forward. This compresses the abdomen between the bottom of the ribs and the upper part of the pelvis, so that the abdomen protrudes, the waist is lost and horizontal skin creases appear on the abdomen.

Naturally, if you are a woman who prides herself on her appearance, these changes are depressing and worrying. You lose your self-esteem. As the spinal curve worsens, everyday activities such as housework, gardening or even sitting for long periods in a chair become uncomfortable. If it progresses to extremes and the curvature brings your rib cage down to meet the pelvic brim, your chest becomes compressed, too, and you find it difficult to breathe. When you try to keep your head up, you get a headache with the effort of stretching and contracting your neck muscles. Your clothes no longer fit, and it is difficult, if not impossible, to find new clothes that do. Add to that a constant fear of falling, now that you can only shuffle around with your eyes fixed on the floor a few feet in front of you, and you can understand why people with vertebral osteoporosis are often very depressed.

## Men with osteoporosis

Much of what has been written so far has been written with women in mind, because most osteoporotic fractures occur in women, but men can develop them too. About 30 per cent of all hip fractures occur in men, and one in eight men over the age of 50 will eventually have a hip fracture. Men's bones are bigger and longer than women's and they have greater total bone mass, but their bone density is similar to that in women, and they lose bone mass steadily from middle age onwards at the same rate as do postmenopausal women.

By the time they are in their fifties, 4 to 6 per cent of men have osteoporosis and around 40 per cent have osteopenia (see Chapter 5). Purely because they have a greater bone mass in their early adult life, men start to have osteoporotic bone fractures around ten years later than women. From age 75 onwards, the numbers of broken hips rise steeply. Their main problem then is recovery. Men don't recover nearly as well or as completely as women from a hip fracture: their death rate within a year of their first fracture is 31 per cent, compared with 17 per cent in women.[1] This is partly because they are older than women at the time of their first break, and partly because they are likely to have other illnesses that make them less able to recover from it.

Half of all men who have had hip fractures continue to have chronic pain at six months and need assistance in walking, and one-third have to move to a nursing home, so that a broken hip in a man is more serious than in a woman of corresponding age. Loss of self-esteem and loss of independence go together, and men who were in good fettle up to the point of the break often lose heart.

As in women, osteoporosis in men can be a complication of long-term steroid use, and of declining hormone levels. A less well-known fact is that men produce oestrogens, obviously to a much lesser degree than testosterone, and that loss of oestrogens as the sex hormone output diminishes can cause osteoporosis in men just as it does in women. No-one has yet promoted oestrogen replacement in men as an answer!

Probably more important for men as causes of osteoporosis are smoking and drinking. Until recent years, men have smoked a lot more than women. Tobacco, as mentioned earlier, interferes with the body's ability to absorb calcium and may well have a direct effect on bones, encouraging bone mineral loss. Heavy-smoking men are much more likely to develop osteoporosis than non-smoking women who have maintained their oestrogens.

Another powerful promoter of osteoporosis in men is excess alcohol. Alcohol, like tobacco, is directly toxic to bone growth. It is also linked to poor eating habits, decreased exercise and a propensity to falling over! So men who drink too much not only have liver and brain problems to contend with, they also face the problems of bone loss.

Most of the guidelines on recognizing and screening for osteoporosis have been drawn up with women in mind, but men deserve a mention too. So any man who has unexpectedly broken a limb in a minor fall should be investigated for osteoporosis with a DXA scan. Men who have lost more than 1.5 inches in height, or whose lower ribs are coming close to the pelvis, need to have spinal X-rays to identify fractures. Like women, if their DXA scan shows a T score of –2.5, men need treatment to strengthen their bones. Their medical treatment is fundamentally the same as for women.

For both men and women with osteoporosis, the aim of the next section of the book is to help you to avoid fractures. You can do much yourself, and your doctors can do the rest with the correct mix of modern treatments.

# 7

# Helping yourself (1) – supplements

Now that you have been given the diagnosis of osteoporosis, your first priority is to do as much as you can to regain the bone density you have lost. You cannot do that without eating correctly. Good nutrition is essential to strong bones, but do we know, exactly, what is the best nutrition for them? For example, many people equate good eating habits and better health with vitamin and mineral supplements. Is this correct? What is the evidence that supplements improve bone strength and prevent broken bones? Is simply eating the right things just as effective?

## Calcium and vitamin D – together

Traditionally, doctors and nutritionists have placed the main emphasis on calcium and vitamin D, either as dietary supplements or in food. Are they enough? It seems unlikely. In May 2005, *The Lancet* published a study of 5,292 people aged 70 or older. Before being admitted to the trial they had all recovered with good mobility after a bone fracture caused by osteoporosis. Half received vitamin D and calcium, and half placebo (a 'dummy' medication).[1] In the following two to five years (the time depended on when each patient joined the study) there were similar numbers of second fractures in the two groups. The authors, doctors from 21 British hospitals, concluded that 'The findings do not support routine oral supplementation with calcium and vitamin D3 either alone or in combination for the prevention of further fractures in previously mobile elderly people.'

It is a disappointing conclusion for everyone involved in osteoporosis, patients and medical staff alike. However, the results aren't as clear-cut as they seem. By two years after starting their tablets, only 2,886 were still taking their tablets. Obviously no blame for this lack of compliance with the rules of the trial can be attached to the 451 who had died in the interim, but 1,955 had stopped taking the tablets – calcium/vitamin D or placebo. More people taking the calcium than the placebo tablets stopped, mainly because of stomach upsets.

That means that if we doctors have to rely on our patients taking calcium supplements every day to prevent osteoporosis, we will be disappointed. Half of you will stop taking the medicines because either they are too much bother or they upset you. And if there is no added benefit, in terms of preventing future fractures, to be had from swallowing calcium tablets, why should you – if you have had a fractured wrist, for example – bother to take them? It seems that we may have to look for extra ways to help ourselves in the battle against osteoporosis.

In the past when we have been advising patients on osteoporosis, we have perhaps concentrated too much on calcium and vitamin D. In July 2003, Beth Kitchin and Sarah Morgan, of the University of Alabama, reviewed the present status of research into nutrition in osteoporosis.[2] Their first conclusion is that although calcium supplements have been shown to decrease bone loss and risk of fracture (except in women many years after the menopause), the increase in bone density is much higher when the supplement is used along with 'antiresorptive' medicines. These will be described later, but for the moment it is enough to explain that they stimulate osteoblasts rather than osteoclasts, and are mainly in the class of drugs known as 'bisphosphonates'. Calcium alone, Kitchin and Morgan write, is unlikely to produce 'full osteoporosis benefits' in patients with low bone mineral density.

Vitamin D supplements, too, turn out to be as complicated as calcium. Vitamin D, as explained earlier, increases the absorption of calcium from the gut and reduces its excretion through the kidneys, so raising the levels of calcium in the blood in two ways. We know a lot about vitamin D and calcium, but the different national authorities (such as Australia, France, the United Kingdom and the United States) still don't agree on how much vitamin D we need to prevent osteoporosis.

## Parathyroid hormone

One of the problems is that there is a complicating factor in the system – parathyroid hormone. Parathyroid hormone is secreted, as explained earlier, by the parathyroid glands in the neck. The higher the blood parathyroid hormone level, the more the balance in bone veers towards loss of mineral, rather than building it up. The aim of calcium and vitamin D supplements is to suppress parathyroid hormone secretion – this will enhance the deposit of calcium into bone, and strengthen it.

Theoretically, giving vitamin D and calcium together may not suppress parathyroid hormone production, but giving them at different times may do so.[3] J. Y. Reginster and colleagues' study showed that separating calcium and vitamin D supplements by six hours was the best way to suppress parathyroid hormone, and gives the best chance for them to work together to improve bone strength. The study also showed that as the amount of calcium we take in increases, the proportion of it that we absorb decreases, so there is an upper limit of calcium intake beyond which there is no extra benefit.

## Vitamin D alone

What about giving vitamin D without the calcium supplement? That, too, has been looked at. The common way to add vitamin D to our diet is to swallow cod liver oil, mostly in capsules, as the drink itself is unpleasant to swallow day after day. Norwegians have a plentiful source of cod liver oil around their shores, so it doesn't come as a surprise that Norwegian doctors are in the forefront of cod liver oil research. H. E. Meyer and colleagues gave 1,144 Norwegian nursing-home residents either extra vitamin D as cod liver oil capsules or similar-looking and similar-tasting placebo capsules for two years.[4] At the close of the trial, there were similar numbers of hip fractures in the two groups. The vitamin D supplement on its own did not protect the patients against osteoporotic fractures.

## Other mineral and vitamin supplements – who needs them?

We know that minerals and vitamins apart from calcium and vitamin D are important to bone health, but do we get enough of them from what we normally eat? If you have osteoporosis, will taking multinutrient supplements over and above normal eating make a difference?

The answer to that question will come as a shock to the tens of thousands of people who swallow these supplements every day. C. Jensen and colleagues did the definitive work on this in the United States, home of the vitamin and mineral supplement industry.[5] The study was entitled 'Long-term effects of nutrient intervention on markers of bone remodelling and calciotropic hormones in late-postmenopausal women'.

The Jensen team divided their subjects into three groups, and followed them for three years. One group were given dietary counselling and asked to eat food containing at least 800 mg calcium, and preferably up to 1450 mg calcium, each day. The second group were given daily supplements of calcium (1450 mg) and vitamin D (10 micrograms, or mcg). The third group were given the same supplements plus a 'multinutrient' supplement containing 600 mg magnesium, 15 mg zinc, 120 mg vitamin C, 80 mcg of vitamin K and 3 mg boron. All of these extra nutrients are believed to be important for bone health. You have probably guessed the results. The additional multinutrient supplement made absolutely no difference to the bone mineral densities (BMDs) of the spine, hip or whole body. The three groups ended the trial with the same readings – improved bone density in each group.

The authors concluded that eating 'bone-friendly' foods containing enough calcium is just as effective in protecting bone against osteoporosis as adding calcium and vitamin D as supplements. They stress that adding other multinutrients has no extra benefits.

## Salt and caffeine

What you eat certainly matters. Salt, for example, is a mineral that few people associate in any way with osteoporosis. Yet a high sodium level (salt is sodium chloride) in your bloodstream causes the kidneys to excrete more calcium, thereby possibly 'sucking' more calcium from the bone. The kidneys react in a similar way to excessive caffeine. It isn't yet clear whether these effects are large enough to make a difference to BMD, but if you have osteoporosis it is probably wise to control (but not to cut out) your intake of salt and of caffeine, of which coffee and cola drinks are the main contributors.

## Tea

If there's bad news about caffeine for coffee drinkers, why not turn to tea? We know tea contains caffeine, which doesn't appear to be beneficial for osteoporosis, but it also contains minerals and other substances that have a more positive role in bone health.

The 'good guys' in tea are fluoride and phyto-oestrogens. In 2002, C. Wu and colleagues asked 1,225 Chinese men and women about the type, amount and duration of their tea drinking.[6] They were interested in whether the amount and type of tea they had drunk over the years had made any difference to their bone density. They compared like for like, in that they adjusted their results for sex, age, body mass index (their body weight/height ratio) and lifestyles.

The results were a great advertisement for Chinese tea – whether it was green, oolong or black. The people who had drunk tea daily for more than ten years had significantly denser bones (and therefore much less risk of osteoporotic fracture) than those who were not habitual tea drinkers. The BMD increase was the same for each type of tea.

The authors postulate that several components in tea, apart from the obvious fluoride and plant oestrogens, could help strengthen bones. Which is the main one remains obscure. They add that, whatever it is, it more than counters the potentially adverse effect on bone of the tea's caffeine content. It seems that doctors who warn people with osteoporosis about caffeine in their drinks should temper that advice when the main source of the daily caffeine is tea. Having read the Wu study, I'm impressed by the protective effect of tea and am happy to promote it here.

## Protein

I'm all for plenty of protein in one's food. Bones need protein as well as minerals to keep strong. However, there is an ongoing debate among the nutritionists on just how much protein we need – and on whether or not too much may be harmful, rather than beneficial.

In an article, Dr D. E. Sellmeyer[7] doesn't beat about the bush; he reports that eating too much meat and too few vegetables is a bad combination for people with osteoporosis.

On the other hand, in the same year B. Dawson-Hughes

and S. S. Harris[8] were writing that people who ate the highest amount of animal protein and also took calcium supplements had the greatest BMDs. They had followed 342 older men and women for three years. Those given 500 mg of calcium as calcium malate and 17.5 mcg of vitamin D, and who were also eating the most protein (animal or vegetable), had the strongest bones. Their trial also had people on placebo: there was no relationship between their protein intake and their BMD, perhaps contradicting Dr Sellmeyer.

One of the differences between the Sellmeyer and the Dawson-Hughes groups may have been in the calcium supplements used. Calcium malate is an alkali that causes the kidney to reduce its excretion of calcium, thereby increasing its blood and bone levels. Eating a lot of fruit and vegetables has the same effect.

Drawing my own conclusions from these rather contradictory papers, it would seem sensible to continue to eat well, with plenty of animal and vegetable protein, and fruit and vegetables. If you eat a lot of red meat, it is probably wise to take a calcium supplement as well, and calcium malate is one of the choices.

## Vitamin A supplements – don't take them

One vitamin supplement that you should *not* take if you have osteoporosis is vitamin A. There are three good scientific studies to support this statement, which probably comes as a surprise to most readers. After all, many people look on vitamin A as inextricably linked with vitamin D in its effects, and there are many over-the-counter vitamin manufacturers who combine the two as a health supplement.

Here are the facts about vitamin A. In 1998, H. Melhus and colleagues reported that excessive intake of vitamin A lowered BMD and increased the risk of hip fractures in northern European women.[9] I assume that many of my readers are in that category.

In the famous US Nurses' study,[10] in which 72,337 women were followed for more than 20 years, the nurses who were not on hormone replacement therapy and who took the most retinol (the active form of vitamin A) had the most hip fractures. Eating foods containing beta-carotene (such as carrots and other yellow and red vegetables), which is a 'precursor' of retinol, into which it is converted in the body, did not have the same osteoporosis-inducing effect.

The figures are hard to argue against. Most of the retinol (vitamin A) was consumed in multivitamin tablets: liver was the main source of retinol eaten in their diet. Women who consumed as much as 2,000 mcg per day of retinol in either or both of these ways had double the risk of fracture of women whose intakes were under 500 mcg per day. The current recommended daily dose of retinol for women is 700 mcg – which may be too high if you have osteoporosis. There is an easy way round this. Rather than taking retinol in pills, eat beta-carotene, but not as a vitamin pill. Consume it the way it was meant to be eaten, in vegetables. Then your body converts what it needs into vitamin A, and it does not raise the risk of fracture.

If that wasn't enough bad news about vitamin A supplements, there is another blow to its proponents: men, like women, react badly to extra vitamin A. In a study into which 2,322 men aged 49 to 51 were enrolled, then followed for 30 years, blood levels of retinol, but not beta-carotene, were strongly linked to fractures.[11] The correlation was very close, with the fracture rate rising by 26 per cent for each standard deviation increase in serum retinol.

It is difficult to persuade people that a vitamin supplement might actually do harm, and even increase their risk of a fracture, especially when the health pages in today's women's magazines (and in men's, too) continually extol the virtues of vitamins and so-called natural food supplements. Vitamins are not magic and are meant to be eaten as a component of food. Once you start swallowing much more than you need, they become a drug, not a vitamin, and you may well lose their benefits as you do so.

## Summarizing on supplements

It is clear that depending simply on taking vitamin and mineral supplements will not improve your chances of avoiding an osteoporosis-induced fracture, and in the case of vitamin A may even worsen them. There is good reason to take extra vitamin D and calcium (though probably at different times of the day), but even for them there is little evidence that on their own your bone density and risk of fracture will both improve. You need something extra, such as the bisphosphonates mentioned earlier, and you need good overall nutrition. The best way to get that is by adopting high-quality eating habits. I don't use the word 'diet' here because it has medical connotations. What you eat is part of your everyday living for the rest of your life: if you look upon it as a diet there are connotations of having to comply with it out of necessity, and the suggestion that some day you may be able to revert to your old ways. If this is in the background of your mind, then it will be only too easy to give up and revert to your old eating habits, and that is not an option for you.

# 8

# Helping yourself (2) – food

This is the most comforting chapter for anyone with osteoporosis. The simple message is that good food is good for you. The aim is to eat a wide variety of foods, especially those that contain vitamin D and calcium, and it just so happens that most of them are tasty and easy to eat. The following list gives foods rich in calcium and vitamin D.

| Calcium-rich | Vitamin D-rich |
|---|---|
| Dairy produce: milk, cheese, butter | Fatty fish: mackerel, sardines, pilchards, herring, halibut, trout, salmon, tuna |
| Eggs | Dairy produce |
| Bread | Vitamin-enriched foods: bread, cereals |

Start by putting on your daily menu plenty of plants that are full of high-quality proteins, such as beans (even baked beans), nuts, seeds and wholegrains. Eat oily fish several times a week, such as sardines, mackerel, pilchards, trout, salmon and tuna. Ring the changes from one to another so that you don't get bored. Cook them in oil, or even with a little butter.

Dive into the fruit bowl every day, and make sure that every meal contains fresh vegetables. They help make your body chemistry a little more alkaline (rather than acid) and that helps drive minerals into bones.

Dairy products are good for you, too. Milk, yogurt and cheese are full of calcium. If you have heart problems and have been warned off milk because of its fat content, then drink semi-skimmed milk. Skimming only removes the fat, not the calcium. There is calcium in bread, too, especially in white bread, because white bread flour has calcium added to it.

The only bad news is to avoid caffeine-containing drinks (except the tea mentioned in the previous chapter), which means going for decaffeinated coffee and avoiding cola. Don't take extra salt in your food – banish the salt cellar from the table, and try not to add it in your cooking. Salt reduces your body's ability to absorb and retain calcium. The same goes, sadly, for alcohol. Stick to a small alcoholic drink each day, but certainly no more than one large or two small glasses of wine.

The sun is also good for you. In these days of dire warnings about the terrible changes the sun can produce in your skin, people have forgotten that we northern people get most of our year's supply of vitamin D from our weak, often watery sunshine. Sunlight on our skin causes it to manufacture vitamin D. Even in our British summers, being in the sun for between 15 and 20 minutes a day gives us enough vitamin D to do us a year. This doesn't mean you have to sunbathe. Just being out and about in the sunshine, preferably doing some exercise, in a short-sleeved shirt and shorts is all that's needed.

So far, so good, but what about becoming overweight? Eating so much of so many potentially fattening foods, you may think, may pile on your weight. In fact that's rarely a problem, partly because few overweight people are osteoporotic in the first place, and by the time you have reached the age of osteoporosis your weight is unlikely to change much. You will already know when you have had enough to eat, and simply changing what you eat in the direction of fish, vegetables, fruit and dairy products is unlikely to make you overweight. In any case, the next way you can help yourself is to exercise properly, and that will keep you trim and feeling good.

# 9

# Helping yourself (3) – exercise

The correct exercise is just as vital as the food you eat. It has to start young to be really effective in preventing osteoporosis, as this is the time when you pack in the minerals into your bones. By the time you are in your fifties it is more difficult to start exercising again if you have been a couch potato for 30 years (as many of us are), but it is worth it.

Let's get rid of the myths about exercise first. For a start, you can't wear out your bones and joints by exercising. In fact, the reverse is the truth. The more you use your muscles and bones and joints, the stronger they will be. That's true even if you have bones that are brittle, as in osteoporosis. You can start your exercising in the swimming pool to begin with, but as long as you are eating well and taking anti-osteoporotic medicines along with it, the correct sort and amount of exercise can do you nothing but good. It is certainly a major way of preventing broken bones.

I've split up my plan for exercise into two parts – the first for people in their fifties and sixties who want to prevent osteoporosis, and the second for people in their seventies and beyond who already have it and wish to reverse it if possible.

## Exercise plans for the fifties and sixties

You are about to retire or have just retired, and you want to keep healthy. Plan your programme of exercise as meticulously as you do your finances. You don't have any excuse not to exercise, for several reasons:

- You have more time to spare now that pressures of work have eased and your children are up and away.
- You may have the great joy of taking your grandchildren on outings (it is certainly one of the joys of my life).
- You probably have more disposable money than before to spend on healthy activities and food.
- You can, for the first time in your life, be a bit more selfish and make your own health and fitness your priority.

Exercise doesn't just mean walking or running on a treadmill at a gym. Trying to do that for the first time at your age is hardly likely to succeed unless you get others to join with you. It's better to make your dreams a reality – to take the opportunity to travel to places you have always wanted to visit, or to learn new skills, like hill walking, cycling, canoeing, anything that takes your fancy and you would really enjoy doing. The London Marathon may be beyond you, but in most cities today there are athletic clubs that organize shorter fun runs and that welcome older citizens.

Aerobics are good fun as well as good exercise, on land as well as in a swimming pool. Remember that one of your motives is to strengthen your bones, so by all means do pool aerobics, but exercise on a solid floor as well. Exercising entirely in water avoids weight-bearing, and weight-bearing is essential if you are to strengthen your bones.

## Exercise plans for the seventies and older with osteoporosis

Hardly any two people in their seventies are alike in their ability to exercise. Some people seem to age faster than others at this stage of life, but much depends on how willing you are to keep up your physical fitness and your outgoing outlook on life. If you haven't exercised for some time and are fearful of perhaps breaking a bone, start slowly and work up. Begin by exercising for five to ten minutes three times a day, and build it up slowly over weeks.

Even at your age and with osteoporosis, as long as you are taking treatment for it, you shouldn't worry that exercise will break a bone spontaneously. Exercise quickly starts to improve your BMD and make you fitter and stronger.

If you wish, start your exercising in water. There are plenty of classes for older citizens at local swimming pools where you can indulge in aerobics with others like you. The camaraderie is wonderful and you will both make new friends and discover new opportunities to take exercise. That may range from walking together to the shops to taking holidays together. A new life can begin at 70 for anyone with the right outlook.

As you exercise, aim to build up your flexibility and your endurance, but don't overdo it. Don't exercise too long or too intensely, and take at least two days a week off, to rest your muscles and joints and allow them to recover. If you are a young 70, then the rules above for the fifties and sixties apply to you, too.

If you are depressed and tired and think that exercise is not for you, think again. Do give it a try. Regular exercise can help you sleep better, get your figure in trim, make you feel younger and well, and help you lose any unwanted pounds. Your self-esteem will shoot up and you will feel ready for anything. It is worth a try. Sitting around at home watching television is not an alternative worth considering. Finally, the exercise will be a big step in increasing your BMD, and will help you avoid a broken wrist or hip or a collapsed vertebra. You will be surprised by how young you will feel, and by how your friends appreciate the new you.

If you are a smoker, however, none of this advice will be of any value to you if you continue your tobacco habit. Nicotine, carbon monoxide and the many tarry substances in cigarette smoke are more than enough to counterbalance any advantage you gain from your new lifestyle. You must stop smoking. The next chapter is for you: it is a desperate effort to persuade you to stop, and gives the reasons in graphic detail.

# 10

# Helping yourself (4) –
# stopping smoking

Every study on osteoporosis has shown that smokers have poorer
bone mineral density than non-smokers. It is abundantly clear
why this is so. The chemicals from smoke interfere with the
bowel wall cells that absorb calcium and other minerals. They
interfere, too, with the liver's ability to produce active vitamin
D from the beta-carotene that is its precursor in our food. They
probably poison the osteoblasts that build up our bones, so that
the balance in bone metabolism swings from building it up to
breaking it down. That should be enough for any smoker with
osteoporosis to stop at once, but I have been a doctor too long
to be fooled. Smoking is such a powerful addiction that these
few facts are not enough for most addicts. So this chapter gives
you the full blast. If you are still able to light up after reading it,
you may as well discard this book and resign yourself to further
fractures and considerable difficulties in the future. If you stop
now, you can look forward to a much healthier and much more
enjoyable old age.

How, exactly, does smoking harm you? Tobacco smoke contains carbon monoxide and nicotine. Carbon monoxide poisons
the red blood cells, so that they cannot pick up and distribute
much-needed oxygen to the organs and tissues, including the
heart muscle. Carbon monoxide-affected red cells (in the 20-a-
day smoker, nearly 20 per cent of red cells are carrying carbon
monoxide instead of oxygen) are also stiffer than normal, so
that they can't bend and flex through the smallest blood vessels.
The gas also directly poisons the heart muscle so that it cannot

contract properly and efficiently, thereby delivering a double whammy of damage to it.

Nicotine causes small arteries to narrow, so that the blood flow through them slows. It raises blood cholesterol levels, thickening the blood and promoting degeneration in artery walls. Both nicotine and carbon monoxide encourage the blood to clot, multiplying the risks of coronary thrombosis and stroke.

Add to all this the tars that smoke leaves in the lungs, which further reduce the ability of red cells to pick up oxygen, and the scars and damage to the lungs that always in the end produce chronic bronchitis and sometimes induce cancer, and you have a formula for disaster.

## The bald facts about smoking

- Smoking causes more deaths from heart attacks than from lung cancer and bronchitis.
- People who smoke have two or three times more risk of a fatal heart attack than non-smokers. The risk rises with the number of cigarettes smoked.
- Men under 45 who smoke 25 or more cigarettes a day have a 10 to 15 times greater chance of death from heart attack than non-smoking men of the same age.
- About 40 per cent of all heavy smokers die before they reach 65. Of those who reach that age, many are disabled by bronchitis, angina, heart failure and leg amputations, all because they smoked. Only 10 per cent of smokers survive in reasonable health to the age of 75. Most non-smokers reach 75 in good health.
- In the UK, 40 per cent of all cancer deaths are from lung cancer, which is very rare in non-smokers. Of 441 British male doctors who died from lung cancer, only seven had never smoked. Only one non-smoker in 60 develops lung cancer: the figure for heavy smokers is one in six!

- Other cancers more common in smokers than in non-smokers include tongue, throat, larynx, pancreatic, kidney, bladder and cervix cancers.

The very fact that you are reading this book means that you are taking an intelligent interest in your health. So after reading this far, it should be common sense to you not to smoke. Yet it is very difficult to stop, and many people who need an excuse for not stopping put up spurious arguments for their stance. Here are ones that every doctor is tired of hearing, and my replies.

*My father/grandfather smoked 20 a day and lived till he was 75.*

Everyone knows someone like that, but they conveniently forget the many others they have known who died long before their time. The chances are that you will be one of them, rather than one of the lucky few.

*People who don't smoke also have heart attacks.*

True. There are other causes of heart attacks, but 70 per cent of all people under 65 admitted to coronary care with heart attacks are smokers, as are 91 per cent of people with angina considered for coronary bypass surgery.

*I believe in moderation in all things, and I only smoke moderately.*

That's rubbish. We don't accept moderation in mugging, or dangerous driving, or exposure to asbestos (which incidentally causes far fewer deaths from lung cancer than smoking). Younger men who are only moderate smokers have a much higher risk of heart attack than non-smoking men of the same age. The figures are even worse for women.

*I can cut down on cigarettes, but I can't stop.*

It won't do you much good if you do. People who cut down usually inhale more from each cigarette and leave a smaller butt, so that they end up with the same blood levels of nicotine and carbon monoxide. You must stop completely.

*I'm just as likely to be run over in the road as to die from my smoking.*

In the UK about 15 people die on the roads each day. This contrasts with 100 deaths a day from lung cancer, 100 from chronic bronchitis, and 100 from heart attacks, almost all of which are due to smoking. Of every 1,000 young men who smoke, on average one will be murdered, six will die on the roads, and 250 will die from their smoking habit.

*I have to die from something.*

In my experience this is always said by someone in good health. They no longer say it after their heart attack or stroke, or after they have coughed up blood.

*I don't want to be old, anyway.*

We define 'old' differently as we grow older. Most of us would like to live a long time, without the inconvenience of being old. If we take care of ourselves on the way to becoming old, we have at least laid the foundations for enjoying our old age.

*I'd rather die of a heart attack than something else.*

Most of us would like a fast, sudden death, but many heart attack victims leave a grieving partner in their early fifties to face 30 years of loneliness. Is that really what you wish?

*Stress, not smoking, is the main cause of heart attacks.*

Not true. Stress is very difficult to measure and it is very difficult to relate it to heart attack rates. In any case, you have to cope with stress whether you smoke or not. Smoking is an extra burden that can never help, and it does not relieve stress. It isn't burning the candle at both ends that causes harm, but burning the cigarette at one end.

*I'll stop when I start to feel ill.*

That would be fine if the first sign of illness were not a full-blown heart attack from which more than one-third die in the first four hours. It's too late to stop then.

*I'll put on weight if I stop smoking.*

You probably will, because your appetite will return and you will be able to taste food again. But the benefits of stopping smoking far outweigh the few extra pounds you may put on.

*I enjoy smoking and don't want to give it up.*

Is that really true? Is that not just an excuse because you can't stop? Ask yourself what your real pleasure is in smoking, and try to be honest with the answer.

*Cigarettes settle my nerves. If I stopped I'd have to take a tranquillizer.*

Smoking is a prop, like a baby's dummy, but it solves nothing. It doesn't remove any causes of stress, and only makes things worse because it adds a promoter of bad health. And when you start to have symptoms, like the regular morning cough, it only makes you worry more.

*I'll change to a pipe or cigar – they are safer.*

Lifelong pipe and cigar smokers are less prone than cigarette smokers to heart attacks, but have five times the risk of lung cancer and ten times the risk of chronic bronchitis of non-smokers. Cigarette smokers who switch to pipes or cigars continue to be at high risk of heart attack, probably because they inhale.

*I've been smoking for 30 years – it's too late to stop now.*

It's not too late, whenever you stop. The risk of sudden death from a first heart attack falls away very quickly after stopping, even after a lifetime of smoking. If you stop after surviving a heart attack, then you halve the risk of a second. It takes longer to reduce your risk of lung cancer, but it falls by 80 per cent over the next 15 years, no matter how long you have been a smoker.

*I wish I could stop. I've tried everything, but nothing has worked.*

Stopping smoking isn't easy unless you really want to do it. You have to make the effort yourself, rather than think that someone else can do it for you. So you must be motivated. If the next few pages do not motivate you, then nothing will.

## How to stop smoking

You must find the right reason for yourself to stop. For someone with osteoporosis it should surely include that you may feel much better and have far fewer symptoms if you stop, and you will be giving yourself a much better chance of remaining healthy for much longer. But there are plenty of other reasons.

If you are a young adult or teenager who sees middle age and sickness as remote possibilities, and smoking as exciting and dangerous, the best attacks on smoking are the way it makes you look and smell. You can also add the environmental pollution of cigarette ends and the way big business exploits developing nations, keeping their populations in poverty while making huge profits by putting land that should be growing food under tobacco cultivation. Pakistan uses 120,000 acres, and Brazil half a million acres of the richest agricultural land to grow tobacco. And as the multinationals are now promoting their product very heavily to the developing world, no teenager who smokes can claim to be really concerned about the health of the poorer nations. Is this as persuasive an argument for you to stop (or not to start) as any about health or looks?

If you are a more mature woman, looks may be the key. Smoking ages you prematurely, causing wrinkles and giving a pale, pasty complexion. If you smoke you will probably experience the menopause at an early age, even in the mid-thirties, which can destroy your plans to have your family after a career.

For men and older women, the prime motivation is better

health. The statistics for men and women in their sixties who smoke are frightening. More than one-third of smoking men fail to reach pension age.

Let us assume that you are now fully motivated. How do you stop? It is difficult. The best way is to become a non-smoker, as if you have never smoked. You throw away all your cigarettes and decide never to buy or accept another one. Announce the fact to all your friends, who will usually support you. Most people find that they don't have true withdrawal symptoms, provided they are happy to stop. A few become agitated, irritable, nervous and can't sleep at night. But people who have had to stop for medical reasons – say, because they have been admitted to coronary care – hardly ever have withdrawal symptoms.

That strongly suggests that the withdrawal problems are psychological, rather than physical. If you can last a week or two without a smoke, you will probably never light up again. The desire to smoke will disappear as the levels of carbon monoxide, nicotine and tarry chemicals in your lungs, blood, brain and other organs gradually subside.

If you must stop gradually, plan ahead. Write down a diary of the cigarettes you will have, leaving out one or two each succeeding day, and stick to it. Carry nicotine chewing gum, get your doctor to prescribe for you a series of nicotine patches or inhalers if you must, but remember that the nicotine is still harmful. Don't look on it as a long-term alternative to a smoke. If you are having real difficulty stopping, ask your doctor for a prescription of Zyban. You may be offered a two-month course of the drug. It helps, but is by no means infallible.

If you do use aids to stop (others include acupuncture and hypnosis), remember that they have no magical properties. They are a crutch to lean on while you make the determined effort to stop altogether. They cannot help if your will to stop is weak.

Recognize, too, that stopping smoking is not an end in itself. It is only part of your new way of life that includes your new way of eating and exercise, and your new attitude to your future health. And you owe it not only to yourself, but also to your partner, family and friends, because it will help to give them a healthier you for, hopefully, years to come. You are not on your own. More than a million Britons have stopped smoking each year for the last 15 years. Only one in three adults now smoke (fewer than one in 20 doctors). By stopping, you are joining the sensible majority.

Now that you are a non-smoker, you can read on and learn about the current medical treatments for osteoporosis.

# 11

# Today's medical treatments for osteoporosis

Today, new medicines only reach the prescription pad after they have been tested and found to be effective in randomized controlled clinical trials (RCTs). In such trials the patients and the attending doctors do not know which treatments they have been given, and the results are not analysed until the planned trial period is over and enough subjects have been treated. As most of the current treatments for osteoporosis have been introduced in the modern period, they have all been subject to RCTs, and the evidence for them is strong. Osteoporosis has attracted considerable attention from academic and drug industry research teams, and this chapter summarizes their efforts and successes over the last two decades. If you have osteoporosis you can, like family doctors such as myself, be very encouraged by the progress that has been made.

Faced with your osteoporosis, you and your doctor have choices to make together. It can be treated by calcium and vitamin D, bisphosphonates, calcitonin, parathyroid hormone, strontium ranelate or selective oestrogen receptor modulators. I'll explain their actions, their successes and their drawbacks one by one.

## Calcium and vitamin D

Most of the evidence for treating osteoporosis with calcium and vitamin D has been reported in Chapter 7, so it isn't repeated here. The combination remains the standard treatment for osteoporosis and its prevention in the frail elderly. Numerous studies have reported that it improves muscle strength and prevents fractures in older women; others have failed to show significant benefit. On balance the combined treatment is worthwhile, but most doctors would prefer to add a bisphosphonate to the treatment.

In the elderly a daily dose of 1.2 grams of calcium and 800 international units of vitamin D3 is the choice in the UK. Calcium preparations include the carbonate, citrate, gluconate, lactate and phosphate. They are all readily absorbed in the gut and there is little, apart from patient preference on taste and convenience, to choose between them. They may all cause indigestion, so they should be taken with food. Some calcium preparations are combined with vitamin D3 in the same chewable tablet. There is debate about whether this is the best way to ensure that both work well together, or whether they should be taken separately, several hours apart. The general view is that the combined tablet is convenient and it has the advantage of having been used with few problems for many years.

## Bisphosphonates

When they were introduced, bisphosphonates were rightly hailed as wonder drugs. They are 'anti-resorptive agents' in that they slow down the actions of osteoclasts. There is debate about how much effect they have on osteoblasts, with some authors claiming that they also tend to block osteoblastic activity, so that their main action is to slow bone turnover. Others suggest that their anti-osteoclast action is greater than that on the osteoblasts, so that the balance of bone turnover is towards building up bone, rather than breaking it down. Whichever theory is correct, the overall effect is an increase in BMD that has been proven in many clinical trials and confirmed in their use in hundreds of thousands of patients over the last five to ten years.

The first bisphosphonate was etidronate. It has to be given in cycles for 14 days at a time, with an interval of 76 days in which calcium carbonate is given. It can't be given continuously, because there is evidence that if it is, the effect reverses, and the bone starts to de-mineralize. That is why the 76-day interval is chosen: if you try to increase the dose or take it without a break, you can actually make things worse, rather than better, for your bones. However, trials performed at the recommended dose have confirmed that it reduces vertebral and non-vertebral fracture rates in women with osteoporosis. The two newer bisphosphonates, alendronate and risedronate, that have been licensed for osteoporosis in the United Kingdom (there are others in other countries) have gained in popularity because they are easier to take and have been at least as successful in their clinical trials as etidronate. They are taken as a single tablet once a week.

All three bisphosphonates have been shown to improve BMD and to reduce fractures. The evidence for alendronate comes from two main clinical trials. In the first, in 359 women with osteoporosis aged between 60 and 85, the benefit lasted throughout the whole age range.[1] In the second, in 327 women aged from 65 to 91, alendronate significantly increased BMD in the spine and hip: there was no change in the women on placebo.[2]

Risedronate was compared with a placebo in a study of osteoporosis that included 5,445 women aged 70 to 79 with a low BMD but no previous fracture, and 3,886 women over 80 years old who had had at least one broken bone.[3] There were 40 per cent fewer fractures in the younger women taking the drug than in those on placebo. As for those who had already had a fracture, they were looked after so well that too few of them had a second fracture in either group to make analysis meaningful. The jury is still out on whether risedronate will prevent a second fracture in older women.

The trial evidence is so strong for bisphosphonates that it is difficult not to prescribe them for women with low BMD levels and for women with proven osteoporosis and a previous fracture. They should also be made available to men with osteoporosis. Bisphosphonates, like all powerful drugs, have their problems. For example, they can irritate the oesophagus (the tube that carries food from throat to stomach), so they must be given with extreme caution, if at all, to anyone with heartburn or with unexplained indigestion. If you have an oesophageal problem that slows or interferes with swallowing (such as a narrowing, or spasm, a condition called achalasia), or long-standing kidney problems, then you must not take bisphosphonates. It is important, too, that you don't have a low blood calcium level and that you are not vitamin D deficient before starting to take them.

Bisphosphonates also have a host of other side effects. They include stomach pains, diarrhoea or constipation (or the two alternating), flatulence, muscle pains and headaches. Less common, but serious enough to stop people taking them, are rashes, itching, the development of skin sensitivity to light, eye inflammations, nausea and vomiting. There are a few reports of severe allergic reactions to them, including the life-threatening anaphylactic shock.

Their dosages are awkward, too. The once-a-week dose is easily forgotten by people who are usually in their seventies and eighties, so they may need reminding to reserve a time for it on the relevant day. If you are taking one of the three bisphosphonates, do read the instructions carefully: to achieve the maximum absorption of the drug, you must follow them to the letter.

For example, with alendronate (once weekly) you must take the tablet as soon as you rise in the morning. It must be swallowed whole with a full glass of water 30 minutes before food, drink or any other medicines. It is important, too, to remain standing for half an hour after taking it. All these precautions are intended to ensure the full absorption of the drug with as short a contact between drug and oesophagus as possible. The instructions for risedronate (once weekly) are just as complicated, for the same reasons. You are advised to swallow the tablet whole with a full glass of water. If you take it immediately after getting out of bed in the morning, it must be swallowed at least 30 minutes before the first food or drink of the day. If you take it at any other time of the day, you should avoid food or drink for at least two hours before or after it. The manufacturers of risedronate and etidronate advise that you should particularly avoid calcium-containing products such as milk, and iron- and mineral-containing supplements and antacids, within two hours of taking them. They are not to be taken last thing at night or before rising in the morning.

Such instructions may seem odd and awkward, but they have been worked out after research into the best way of delivering the drugs to their target – your bones – and it is best to obey them to the letter. You have the advantage with risedronate and alendronate that they only need to be taken once weekly, so that your daily routine is only altered occasionally. On the other hand, if you forget to take that once-weekly tablet, you will lose the benefit for a whole week, so do make sure that you set aside a particular day a week for taking your medicine, and organize some sort of memory aid to help you. Sticking a large label on the kitchen calendar or beside the medicine cabinet in the bathroom is a start.

Osteoporosis is not the only illness in which the bone density needs to be increased. Women with breast cancer sometimes develop secondary cancers (metastases) in their bones that leave the bones weaker and liable to fracture. In Paget's disease of the bone, cysts form which are sometimes so large that the bone breaks spontaneously. Bisphosphonates are useful in both of these distressing illnesses. Several bisphosphonates are specifically licensed for them, and not for osteoporosis, and can be very effective. For example, within a few days of starting them, people with bone metastases or Paget's disease report very considerable, and sometimes complete, relief of bone pain. The bisphosphonates used for these bone diseases include pamidronate (Aredia), ibandronate (Bondronat), clodronate (Bonefos, Loron), tiludronate (Skelid) and zoledronate (Zometa). Most have to be given by slow intravenous injection, very carefully, to avoid serious side effects.

Two of them have been used outside their licence restrictions ('off-label' in medical parlance) for osteoporosis. Pamidronate has been given to postmenopausal women with osteoporosis who had intolerable side effects with the standard bisphosphonates in two trials. In one study they were given five courses at four-week intervals; in the other they were given three courses. The drug increased their bone density at the hip and the spine, but the trials are too small to tell whether it protected against fractures.

Zoledronate was given at one-year intervals, and even this annual treatment increased bone density in the women. Their bone density measurements increased by around 5 per cent during the treatment period. However, as with pamidronate, there are no data on fractures, and it is not yet recommended for general use in osteoporosis.

## Calcitonin

Calcitonin is a curious hormone, in that it is made in very large amounts by salmon, which need it to control the changes that occur in their bodies during the transfer between salt and fresh water. The calcitonin used in medicine is mainly produced from salmon. We ourselves secrete calcitonin from our thyroid glands in the neck: its purpose is to lower calcium levels in the blood by shifting calcium into the bone, and to block the leaching of calcium from bone back into the blood – an action opposite to that of parathyroid hormone. The two hormones act in unison to keep our calcium levels within strict limits. Obviously, giving calcitonin to someone with osteoporosis will lead to higher calcium levels in the bones and should, in theory, be of considerable benefit.

However, calcitonin isn't easy to make or to give at a standard dose. Being a hormone, it is broken down in the stomach by digestive juices, so it can't be given in the form of a pill. Until recently it was only available as an injection (as Miacalcic), and was restricted to people with abnormally high blood calcium levels, Paget's disease or metastases into bones from breast or prostate cancer.

Now Miacalcic is available as a nasal spray, and it has been granted a licence for prescription to postmenopausal women with osteoporosis. The hormone in the spray is absorbed into the bloodstream through the membranes of the surface of the inside of the nose without having to go through the stomach. It is given as a single spray of 200 units (each spray contains an exact dose) into one nostril, once a day. It must be given with calcium and vitamin D supplements.

As with the bisphosphonates, if you have bone pain (from osteoporosis or other bone diseases) it will ease very quickly after starting on calcitonin, long before it could have any significant influence on your BMD. C. Gennari, writing on the analgesic effect of calcitonin in 2002,[4] found this to be a very striking advantage of the treatment and proposed that the calcitonin releases natural opiates from the brain.

Whatever the mechanism of the immediate pain relief, there is no doubt that, in the long term, calcitonin nasal spray works well in osteoporosis. In a double-blind randomized placebo-controlled trial over five years (clearly very strong evidence) in 1,255 women with already established osteoporosis taking the 200 unit dose by nasal spray, there were 33 per cent fewer new spinal fractures in those receiving the active spray than in those given the placebo.[5] The women on the active treatment also had higher BMD measurements by the end of the trial. Curiously, the treatment did not show any protection against hip fractures. Even though calcitonin is a natural hormone, there are reports of side effects from it, although they are rare. They include nausea, vomiting, diarrhoea, flushing, dizziness, tingling of the fingers, unpleasant taste, rash, abdominal pain and allergic reactions. The spray may cause irritation and small ulcers in the inside of the nostril, so it is advisable to alternate the dose from one nostril to the other each day. It may also cause sinusitis and nosebleeds.

Also, because it is a hormone made from salmon, it is possible for the body to set up antibodies against it, so that it loses its effect. So far there is little evidence of this happening with the salmon preparation: it was more common with the previous calcitonin material that was collected from pigs.

The lack of evidence for protection against hip fractures has made British experts reluctant to recommend calcitonin as a first-line drug for most women with osteoporosis, and the general consensus is that it should be reserved for people who have failed to respond to, or have problems with, bisphospho-nates. However, it is recommended for people with bone pain, particularly in the back, caused by osteoporosis.

## Teriparatide (human parathyroid hormone)

Here is where explanation becomes difficult. We know that calcitonin helps build up bone, and it has the opposite effect to parathyroid hormone. Yet a form of human parathyroid hormone has been licensed – and works well – in osteoporosis. The reason for this is that parathyroid hormone increases the activities of both the osteoclasts and the osteoblasts, making bone turnover faster. If a form of it can be found that tips the balance slightly towards the osteoblasts, so that the overall effect is positive, then it should be effective against osteoporosis.

This is what appears to happen with teriparatide, a 'recombinant' human parathyroid hormone. It is classified as an 'anabolic' hormone (one that builds up tissues). It was approved by the American authorities (the Food and Drug Administration) for osteoporosis in November 2002 and by the UK Committee on Safety of Medicines (CSM) shortly afterwards.

Teriparatide increases bone density, thickens both the cancellous and cortical bone, and blocks the 'suicide' message within old osteoblasts. This last needs a little explanation. Every cell in our bodies has a hidden mechanism for 'committing suicide' within it. The proper name for this is 'apoptosis', and it switches on when the cell is ageing and near the end of its useful life. For some cells, such as some white blood cells, or the cells lining the gut, apoptosis 'turns on' in a few days. For others, such as bone and cartilage cells, apoptosis doesn't occur for months. If the apoptosis message is postponed in a bone cell, it continues to function as a source of strength, so this action of teriparatide is a positive one for people with osteoporosis.

The clinical trials of teriparatide have been comprehensive. One involving 1,637 postmenopausal women with vertebral fractures showed that it increased lumbar spine BMD by 10 per cent and hip BMD by 2.8 per cent.[6] More important, after ten months the risk of a new spinal fracture was reduced by a massive 65 per cent and of other fractures by 54 per cent, and the effect was not affected by age, so that it was as beneficial in the very old as in women in their immediately postmenopausal years. In a comparison between teriparatide and alendronate, the parathyroid hormone produced a 12.2 per cent increase in spinal BMD, compared with a 5.6 per cent increase on the bisphosphonate.[7] Teriparatide increased femoral neck BMD and total body minerals, and decreased non-spinal fractures.

Teriparatide has a drawback, however. It is slower to work than bisphosphonates; it takes between three and six months

longer to start protecting against fractures, so if you are prescribed it, you must be patient.

There is another difficulty. It isn't clear whether you should
take both teriparatide and bisphosphonates together, or whether
they are strict alternatives as treatment. Trial results suggest that
taking both types of drug in combination reduces their overall
effects. In a trial of the two drugs separately or combined in
postmenopausal women, the gains in BMD were lower on the
combination than on either drug alone, with teriparatide producing the best results.[8] The same was found in men.[9]

It seems from these studies that if you are taking teriparatide,
you should probably not also take a bisphosphonate: the
bisphosphonate may partially block teriparatide's beneficial
effect on bone cells. So far, all the evidence comes from studies
of bone density changes: because teriparatide is such a new drug
we may have to wait a year or two before we know exactly how
well it protects against fractures. Logically, it should do so at
least as well as bisphosphonates.

As with the other drugs, side effects have been reported
with teriparatide. They include nausea, heartburn and haemor-
rhoids, although it is difficult to understand how it could have
caused the latter! There are reports of fainting due to postural
hypotension (a fall in blood pressure when moving from lying
or sitting to standing up), breathlessness, depression, dizziness,
an increased desire to pass urine, muscle cramps, sciatica and
increased sweating on the drug.

Teriparatide must be given by a daily injection under the
skin (not into muscle), so that if you are prescribed it you will
need to learn to self-inject. It is prescribed as a single pre-filled
'pen' injector containing 28 doses made up in a total of 3 ml of
fluid, so that the volume of each injection is very small. Most
people find it simple and of little consequence. It is licensed in
the UK for treatment for up to 18 months. This time should be
extended as we learn from experience more about the drug. As

each pen costs £271 it is relatively expensive, and for the time being in the UK general practitioners have been instructed that treatment with it can only be initiated by a specialist. Its expense may restrict its use to people who have failed to improve on other medicines.

## Strontium ranelate

Strontium ranelate is the first of a new class of drugs for osteoporosis. It has two actions: reducing bone resorption and increasing bone formation. The proof of its efficacy in osteoporosis comes from a randomized controlled trial[10] in 649 postmenopausal women with osteoporosis and at least one vertebral fracture. The women showed increases in BMD of 12.7 per cent in the lumbar spine and of 8.6 per cent in the hip after three years of treatment, although part of this increase is owing to the fact that strontium (which is incorporated into the bone by the treatment) has a higher atomic number than, and is therefore heavier than, calcium.

That study showed that there were 41 per cent fewer new vertebral fractures in the women taking strontium ranelate than in the control group. In another study of 5,091 women with osteoporosis, there was a 16 per cent reduction in non-spinal fractures.[11] Even more striking were the results among the 1,977 older women (over 74 years old) in this trial who had very low BMD T scores of more than –3.0: strontium reduced their hip fracture rate by 36 per cent.

Strontium ranelate is prepared in powder form in sachets, which are emptied into water. One should be taken each bedtime at least two hours after eating or taking other medicines, to ensure maximum absorption from the gut. That warning particularly applies to milk and other calcium-containing products, and antacids containing aluminium or magnesium salts. Unlike many of the other drugs for osteoporosis, strontium ranelate does not appear to cause indigestion or heartburn. A few people (in the trials 6.1 per cent, compared to the 3.2 per cent on placebo) reported diarrhoea, but it was short-lived. Other reported side effects, but apparently so far very rare, include venous thrombosis (clots in veins), headache, dermatitis and eczema.

## Raloxifene

Raloxifene is technically a 'selective oestrogen receptor modulator' (SERM). It was developed as part of research into hormone replacement and breast cancer treatments. It has a pro-oestrogenic effect on the bones, but an anti-oestrogen effect on the breast and womb, which makes it attractive as a treatment for osteoporosis since hormone replacement therapy (HRT) has run into trouble. I have devoted the next chapter to the evidence for and against HRT in osteoporosis, but raloxifene is in a different category, and is probably most appropriately mentioned here.

The main study of raloxifene was reported by B. Ettinger and colleagues in 1999.[12] It involved treatment of 7,705 women aged 31 to 80 years with osteoporosis. Raloxifene increased lumbar spine and femoral neck BMD by 2 to 3 per cent, reducing the numbers of vertebral fractures by 30 to 50 per cent, and decreased the proportion of women developing breast cancer. It did not reduce their numbers of hip fractures. Although generally it is not considered as effective as bisphosphonates, it is recommended for younger postmenopausal women with osteoporosis who are considered at high risk of spinal fracture.

SERMs like raloxifene, such as tamoxifen (used for breast cancer), do have two side effects that seriously undermine their use.[13] One is the rise in risk of venous thrombosis (clots in veins) that can embolize (break off and travel) to other parts of the body, especially the lungs. About 8 per cent of women taking raloxifene develop venous thrombosis and leg cramps. If you are taking raloxifene and you develop painful legs (particularly calves and thighs), then see your doctor: it may just be cramps, but you must rule out a thrombosis.

The other problem for raloxifene is that it can cause severe hot flushes and sweats. If you are taking raloxifene you should be aware of these risks, particularly if you are just past your menopause. As raloxifene causes these menopausal symptoms, many doctors refrain from prescribing it to recently postmenopausal women, to avoid making their menopausal discomfort worse. Most doctors wait until five years after the woman's last menstrual period before prescribing it. It is taken as a single 60 mg tablet once daily, and has the advantage of being taken at any time during the day with no need for precautions about taking it separately from other medications or foods.

## Hormone replacement therapy (HRT)

For many years HRT was the preferred choice for most women who needed treatment for and prevention of osteoporosis. By 2002, however, this had changed with the results of the Women's Health Initiative (WHI) study. The change has been so important that a separate chapter is needed to explain it, so it is the subject of Chapter 12.

## Summary of today's treatments for osteoporosis

The aim of this chapter has been to describe in detail the modern treatments for osteoporosis, and to do that it was necessary to give the evidence for each treatment in turn, including the references for the evidence. However, because the sections on each treatment have been so comprehensive, it isn't easy to compare the merits of each treatment at a glance. That's why I am finishing the chapter with a table, taken from the Royal College of Physicians' (RCP) clinical guidelines for prevention and treatment of osteoporosis.[14]

**Table 11.1 The trial evidence for the medical management of osteoporosis**

|  | Vertebral fractures | Non-vertebral fractures | Hip fractures |
|---|---|---|---|
| Calcium + vitamin D | ND | A | A |
| Etidronate | A | B | A |
| Alendronate | A | A | A |
| Risedronate | A | A | A |
| Calcitonin | A | B | B |
| Raloxifene | A | ND | ND |
| Teriparatide | A | A | ND |
| Strontium ranelate | A | A | A |
| HRT | A | A | B |

A  Randomized controlled trials.
B  Trials without controls, or epidemiological (population) studies that have less statistical weight behind them.
ND  These trials have not shown a reduction in fractures.

Table 1 is a comparison of the effects of drug treatments on the incidence of vertebral, non-vertebral (mostly wrist) and hip fractures, and the quality of the evidence for them. The teriparatide and strontium ranelate rows have been added to the original RCP table because they were not available at the time (2000) it was published.

The table shows that general practitioners now have a widening range of effective treatments for osteoporosis. Bisphosphonates are the standard, but teriparatide and strontium ranelate are recent additions that promise well. Calcitonin, too, will find its place.

In January 2005, the National Institute of Clinical Excellence (NICE) published its appraisal of the treatments of osteoporosis. Its recommendations will surely influence your doctor's choice from the list of drugs in the table. Nevertheless, doctors jealously guard their independence in what they prescribe, and you will certainly have your say, too, on what you wish to take for your bones. Here is the current NICE guidance for GPs in England, Wales and Northern Ireland. The Scottish guidelines are similar.

Bisphosphonates are recommended as treatment options for the secondary prevention of osteoporotic fractures in susceptible postmenopausal women. In women who cannot take a bisphosphonate or who have suffered a fragility fracture despite treatment for a year and whose bone mineral density declines below the pre-treatment level, the selective oestrogen receptor modulator raloxifene is an alternative. The parathyroid hormone fragment teriparatide is recommended for women over 65 years who cannot take a bisphosphonate (or in whom bisphosphonate has failed to prevent a fracture) and have:

- either an extremely low bone mineral density
- or a very low bone mineral density, suffered two or more fractures, and have other risk factors for fractures (e.g. body mass index below 19 kg/m$^2$, premature menopause, prolonged immobility, history of maternal hip fractures under the age of 75 years).

Doctors don't need to follow NICE slavishly: you and your doctor will surely discuss what is best for you as an individual, and come to a mutually appropriate conclusion about your treatment.

# 12

## Hormone replacement therapy (HRT) – do you wish to take it?

Until 2002 many millions of women worldwide were taking hormone replacement therapy (HRT) with no qualms or worries. They saw the continuation of their hormonal life, with oestrogen and progestogen, as a natural way to keep feeling young. HRT's prime purpose was to help women during and after the menopause to avoid the symptoms of hormone withdrawal, the main ones being hot flushes and sweats, depression and tension, and drying and shrinking of the vagina so that sex becomes difficult at a time when women can really appreciate the lack of need for contraception. With it came the supposed bonuses of protection against heart disease and osteoporosis.

Then the Women's Health Initiative (WHI) study burst the HRT bubble.[1] It showed that for every 10,000 women taking HRT for a year, there were five fewer hip fractures, four fewer bowel cancers, but seven more heart attacks, eight more strokes, eight more pulmonary embolisms (clots broken off from thromboses elsewhere to lodge in a lung) and eight more invasive breast cancers than among 10,000 women who were not HRT users. The authors concluded that the overall health risks from taking HRT were higher than the benefits in protection against osteoporosis.

Doctors and the women themselves were deeply affected by the results, which were wholly unexpected. Taken as figures per 10,000 women each year, the changes affect only a very small number of women, but if they are extrapolated to the millions of women who have been taking HRT for many years, then the treatment was apparently causing several hundred early deaths per year in Britain, and many more than that in the United States. That is why doctors in Britain now limit their HRT, prescribing strictly for a six-month period only for women with severe menopausal symptoms.

Nevertheless, if you are a woman who feels awful without her HRT and feels good on it, you can make the choice, once all the risks are explained to you, to continue with it. Many women make that choice in full understanding of the extra risks, and I have no quarrel with them. My own feeling is that they should only do so on the basis that the HRT is considerably improving their quality of life, physically, socially and sexually. It has been proven to reduce bone fractures in older women, but it is no more effective than, say, bisphosphonates in doing so. So if you choose to continue with HRT beyond six months, it must be for a reason other than preventing or treating osteoporosis. The fact that it helps in osteoporosis is a secondary consideration for you.

# 13

# Non-drug treatments

The last two chapters may have given the impression that the only proven treatments for osteoporosis involve prescription drugs. This isn't so. They are important, but there are other ways in which anyone with osteoporosis can be helped, among them surgery, hip protectors, posture training supports, and balance and exercise training.

## Surgery

Surgery is reserved for people whose vertebrae have collapsed, and for whom the resulting curvature of the lower spine ('kyphosis') is painful and compressing the internal organs of the abdomen. The two operations are vertebroplasty and kyphoplasty. In both operations a polymer called PMMA is injected into the 'bodies' – the centres – of collapsed vertebrae, restoring as much as possible the original shape. Kyphoplasty has the additional aim of inserting a balloon into the vertebral body to restore some height by expanding the collapsed area of bone.

Both have had good results. I. H. Lieberman and colleagues[1] reported on 70 kyphoplasties in 30 patients with osteoporotic compression vertebral fractures. The patients regained 47 per cent of their lost height, and their pain scores (a measure of pain severity) and their physical function both improved greatly. In another report on 55 kyphoplasties in 18 patients, the patients regained more than one-third of their lost height, and the surgery led to improved scores for pain, physical and social function, and vitality.[2] Kyphoplasty also improved pain 'dramatically' and helped straighten kyphosis in another series of 15 patients.[3] The authors concluded that restoring vertebral shape and height was more beneficial if the patients were given a month of conservative care (mainly rest) before the operation.

## Hip protectors

Hip protectors are usually made of polypropylene, and worn on the side of the hip to protect the bone in a fall. In the largest trial, involving 1,409 women and 392 men known to be at high risk of falling, those who wore the hip protectors had fewer fractures than those allocated to no hip protection.[4] The authors calculated that 411 people had to wear hip protectors for one year to prevent one fracture: the corresponding figure for five years was eight people.

This is a huge contribution to preventing hip fractures, but it has the drawback that most people stop wearing the protectors after a fairly short time. Trial reports vary, but the numbers in each study who continue to wear their protectors range from only 35 to 48 per cent. A main problem is that the protectors are difficult to manipulate because most are in the form of under-wear that is difficult to remove, particularly for older people who already have problems with balance and dexterity. The problem rises steeply if the person has difficulty in controlling urinary continence.

On the other hand, some people find that the hip protectors give them self-confidence, and elderly women, in particular, find that when wearing them they not only have less fear of falling, they actually fall less often because they are less frightened by the thought of moving around their home.[5] The less fear they have, the more co-ordinated they become.

## Posture training supports

These are lightweight supports that are worn as a backpack, loaded with weights of just under 1 kg (2 lb). They are worn by people with kyphoses caused by vertebral fractures. The supports not only ease pain, they also help to strengthen the back muscles when used with an exercise programme. Improving the strength of the long muscles that extend the spine (arching it backwards) reduces kyphosis and prevents fractures in older women and younger women with osteoporosis due to oestrogen deficiency (such as after the ovaries have been removed or an early menopause). Unfortunately there are no randomized trial results to confirm that such supports produce a sustained benefit, so there is still doubt about their true usefulness.

## Balance and exercise training – t'ai chi

Anyone who has visited China or Korea could not have failed to be impressed by the balancing ability of the older citizens who gather in local parks to take part in the slow exercises of t'ai chi. American researchers S. L. Wolf and colleagues of the Atlanta FICSIT Group[6] found the t'ai chi exercises reduced the risk of falling by 47.5 per cent, a huge saving in probable fractures. T'ai chi appears to improve balance when patients find themselves in difficult conditions, such as poor lighting, uneven floors and pavements, and noisy and crowded places.

Standard exercise training does increase bone mineral density, but it hasn't been proven to drive down fracture numbers. Postmenopausal women who wore weighted vests and took part in jumping exercises three times a week for 32 weeks each year for five years did improve their hip BMD level. Men who exercised vigorously and regularly had fewer hip fractures than those who preferred to remain sedentary, but there is good evidence that you have to continue exercising briskly if you wish to maintain your improvement in bone density.[7]

It is clear that we need both balance and bone strength. Daily t'ai chi exercises go a long way to providing both, and seem at least as effective as any other treatment in preventing falls, which is a prime aim for anyone with osteoporosis. Most towns offer t'ai chi exercises for their older citizens, as the practice is growing. I've tried it myself and, much to my surprise, I found it challenging and very pleasant. The discipline of slow, deliberate movement is one that I thoroughly recommend, not just for osteoporosis but for a good toning-up exercise at the beginning of every day.

It is clear from this that taking on the challenge of osteoporosis needs a mixture of medication, exercise and the right attitude of mind to see your treatment through. The drugs can help, as can the exercises and the protectors, but in the final analysis the effort must come from you. If you don't take your treatment (as many people don't), and if you become a couch potato (as many people do), and if you can't be bothered wearing your protection (as most people can't), then none of what you have read so far will do you any good. Please be keen to help yourself, and you will find that you will feel better, and almost certainly avoid those dreaded fractures.

# 14

## Future treatments

Most people who are given prescriptions for drugs to prevent fractures stop taking them after a few months. After a year, only a small minority are still taking them, and many of those who have stopped are at very high risk of fractures. Although the drugs are effective, many people find taking them every day too much of a chore, or even that their side effects are intolerable. It is of little use having a treatment that works if too few people can tolerate taking it for long enough to make a difference.

This is a powerful reason for continuing research into better-tolerated drugs for osteoporosis. But where are they to come from? Just think what might happen if a drug that costs a few pennies, causes no serious side effects and has been around for so many years that any problems with it are well known and easily overcome, was found to be effective in promoting bone growth.

### Nitrates

It is just possible that we have such a group of drugs. They are called 'nitrates', and have been used for years in heart disease to open coronary arteries. Dr Sophie Jamal of the University of Toronto has been studying nitrates and bone growth for several years. In her trial of 144 postmenopausal women with osteoporosis given a simple nitrate, Dr Jamal found that, after three months, their bone breakdown decreased by 47 per cent and their bone formation increased by 20 per cent.[1] These are better figures than the most effective bisphosphonates can give.

Dr Jamal is planning further studies of the nitrate isosorbide mononitrate in men and women with osteoporosis. She says, rightly, that nitrates don't cause breast cancer, like oestrogens, or heartburn, like bisphosphonates, and as they have been used for over a hundred years they have a better-known safety profile than almost any other drug, and certainly more than the other drugs in use for osteoporosis.

How nitrates work remains a problem. Curiously, it may matter that they are not taken every day. Dr Jamal found that women who have taken nitrates as needed for chest pain, but not every day, have higher hip and heel BMDs than those who do not take them at all, or than women who take them at least every day.

We will have to wait and see. Some years ago statin drugs were being promoted as possible drugs for osteoporosis because they were thought to raise BMD in animals. They do not do so in human beings. Dr Jamal's work will have to be confirmed by other groups of researchers before the nitrate theory is accepted.

## Ultra-low dose oestrogen

We have known for years that standard doses of oestrogen improve BMD and lower the risk of fractures, but, as discussed in Chapter 12, they were abandoned when the extra risks of breast cancer and heart disease outweighed the benefit for bones. The researchers are not giving up, however, on the oestrogen story. There is reason to believe that ultra-low doses of oestrogen, in the form of oestradiol, may help the bones without raising the risks of other diseases. Already in research is a patch that will deliver through the skin the tiny dose of 0.014 mg of oestradiol daily. When used for two years it does increase bone density significantly more than a placebo. It will be some years, however, before the negative effects can be disproved.

## Once-a-year treatment

Osteoporosis treatment may even be given only once a year. A once-a-year dose of the bisphosphonate zoledronic acid has been in trials for some years. It is already licensed for the treatment of certain bone cancers and in patients with hypercalcaemia (too much calcium in the blood). It has already been shown to improve bone growth in osteoporosis, an effect that is similar whether it is given every three, every six or every twelve months. Zoledronic acid is now undergoing very large clinical trials to find how safe the once-a-year dose is, and whether it keeps its effectiveness after several years. A once-a-year injection would not only avoid the difficulties patients have with continuing to take their treatment, it would also mean far fewer visits by patients to their doctors for follow-up – something that both will appreciate.

Another new bisphosphonate in osteoporosis trials is ibandronate, with a schedule of one injection every four weeks.

## More SERMS? And others?

Teriparatide (see Chapter 11) is only the first of the anabolic hormones under study for their use in osteoporosis. In 2003, M. J. Horwitz and colleagues of the University of Pittsburgh[2] reported on the use of a substance related to teriparatide called 'parathyroid hormone-related protein' (PTHrP). This attaches itself to the same bone cells as parathyroid hormone and induces bone growth. In this initial trial the women taking PTHrP showed similar increases in bone density to those taking teriparatide, without its side effects.

According to the lead investigator of the PTHrP trials, Dr Andrew Stewart, it is going into larger trials to determine its correct dose and to establish further its value in men and women with osteoporosis. He added that there are other similar potential treatments within this class of proteins. Be prepared to hear about drugs called 'bone morphogenic proteins' that will not only strengthen bones but even re-shape them into their previous structure. Also in the frame for development are drugs that Dr Stewart calls 'sclerosin-like' which mimic substances we produce naturally that harden bone, and molecules which mimic receptors for the fats that are needed to build up the material between normal bone cells. These are 'low density lipo-protein receptor agonists'. They may be a few years away from the prescription pad, but Dr Stewart is very hopeful that they will bring good results for future osteoporosis sufferers.

## Organizing new treatments

Once we have these new treatments, for how long should we give them to individual patients? The answer to that question is still a matter of debate among the experts. The best evidence so far is that it is enough to give treatment for three or four years. After that it may be wise to stop and watch patients to see if the bone density deteriorates again. The current data suggest that the effects of three or four years of anti-osteoporosis treatment last for several years after they are stopped. Until we have had much longer trials than those already published, we can't be sure that long-term treatment is needed, and it may even be harmful.

There is an argument for performing bone mineral density scans (DXAs) routinely in women over 50 to see if they are par-ticularly at risk of osteoporotic fractures. Although the fractures do not occur until most women are 70 or over, treatment in their fifties may be the best way of avoiding them.

This leads to the argument about whether or not women with osteopenia (a bone density level below the normal, but not enough to diagnose osteoporosis) should be treated before they become osteoporotic. On balance the experts say they should not. According to one of these experts, Dr Nelson Watts of the

University of Cincinnati, a 30-year-old woman with a BMD T score of −1.1 has normal bones and does not need a medical-sounding label to worry her for the next 40 years. Yet she may well be diagnosed as osteopenic. However, a 74-year-old woman who has a T score of −2.3 and has already had two fractures has true osteoporosis, but will be diagnosed as osteopenic, not osteoporotic, purely from her bone score. She needs intensive treatment.

This leaves doctors in general practice like myself in a quandary: do we make the diagnosis on the DXA score, or on the patient's history? I am for using the patient's history as the basis, and reinforcing the diagnosis with the DXA score. If she has signs and symptoms of the illness, and a T score that suggests she only has osteopenia, I will treat her as if she is osteoporotic. I am sure my colleagues here in the UK will do the same.

# 15

# Questions and answers

I have been writing a 'question and answer' column in various British newspapers since the early 1980s, and questions about osteoporosis have featured regularly in the letters sent to me. Here is a typical sample, chosen to illustrate the fears that many people have about this disease. I hope they help to reassure you.

> Q: *My mother and her sister both developed osteoporosis in their seventies, and seemed to shrivel away over only a few years. Could I go like that? I'm 58 and my periods stopped seven years ago.*

A: Osteoporosis is very common, so even if there were no inherited link, you would still be at risk of developing it. But your early life was probably very different from that of your mother and aunt. You probably ate different food and exercised in a different way, and your early adult life was probably very different from theirs, too. However, there is no denying that with two close relatives with osteoporosis, you are at a statistically higher risk than others of developing it. With that family history your doctor will be happy to check your bone density. If it is normal, you can be reassured. If it is low you will be offered treatment to prevent any further deterioration, and even to build up your bone mass again. You will be looked after so that you can't deteriorate in the same way as the earlier generation of women in your family.

> Q: *I have osteoporosis of the spine, which has caused me to lose two or three inches in height. I'm told that my vertebrae have collapsed. Does that mean I could become paralysed?*

A: No. The collapse occurs in the middle of the spinal bone, not near the spot where the nerves emerge from the spinal cord. That's why osteoporosis rarely causes sciatica, which is much more likely to be the result of a bulging 'disc' (the rubbery cartilage between the vertebrae that acts as a shock absorber) pressing on the nerves, rather than a bone problem. So don't be unduly worried. If you do develop sciatica, see your doctor, who may then investigate for a disc difficulty.

*Q: I'm on tamoxifen for breast cancer. I understand that it is an 'anti-oestrogen' that blocks the oestrogen receptors on cancer cells in the breast and shuts down their activity. As oestrogens in the form of HRT are good for osteoporosis, won't tamoxifen make my osteoporosis worse?*

A: No. Tamoxifen is anti-oestrogenic when it reaches the breast cancer cells, but it has an entirely different action on bone cells, where it even protects against bone loss. It is a SERM (see Chapter 11), in the same class of drugs as raloxifene, so in fact it should lower your chances of developing osteoporosis.

*Q: My aunt is in her eighties and has already lost a lot of height from spinal osteoporosis. She is almost bent double with the spinal curvature. Is there any point in giving her anti-osteoporosis treatment at this late stage? Would it do any good now she is so badly affected?*

A: There are good reasons to start her on treatments such as bisphosphonates. They can't reverse the fractures that have already occurred, but they can prevent further deterioration and more fractures. If she is otherwise physically and mentally fit, she might even be able to benefit from corrective surgery, such as the kyphoplasty or vertebroplasty mentioned in Chapter 13. Today's anaesthetists and surgeons can work wonders, even in the very elderly, provided her general health is up to the operation.

*Q: To be frank, I don't really have many symptoms of osteoporosis, but I'm told because of my early menopause and tests showing a low bone density that I should take treatment. I have been on a bisphosphonate for some months now, and don't feel any different – worse or better –*

*from my normal healthy self before I started on it. Do I really need to
take the treatment, and if so how do I know that it is working?*

A: Your bisphosphonate will increase your bone density, but
you have no internal mechanism that can make that change
obvious to you – it doesn't register in your consciousness. You
benefit from it by not having a fracture – and you will never
know whether or not the treatment has prevented one. You will
have to accept that your risk of breaking a bone must have been
high for your doctor to have started you on treatment, and that
every year that passes without a fracture is a bonus that may
or may not have been due to it. In about two to three years a
second bone density measurement may give you numbers by
which you can calculate your new risk of a fracture. My guess
is that if you stay on the drug that will be smaller, even though
you are older. If you do not take it, your risk will climb steadily
as you grow older.

*Q: My osteoporosis gives me a constant pain in my back, which hasn't
eased much since I started on treatment. Does that mean that the treatment isn't working, or is the back pain caused by something else?*

A: Treatments like bisphosphonates or vitamin D and calcium do
not directly affect pain, so that you could be slowly improving
your bone density while the pain persists, even if the pain is
truly the result of your osteoporosis. If that is the case, it may
take several months, or even a year or two, before the bone is
strong enough for the pain to be fully relieved. However, low
back pain is very common in people without osteoporosis, and
is often the result of muscle cramps due to poor posture and
lack of stretching and exercise (see *Overcoming Back Pain*, Dr Tom
Smith, Sheldon Press, 2003). So tell your doctor about the pain,
and you may be put on other treatment for it alongside that for
your osteoporosis.

*Q: My 85-year-old mother has had three broken bones (two wrists
and a hip) because of severe osteoporosis. She was put on alendronate,*

*but felt nauseated after taking it. She wouldn't take any more, despite being persuaded that the nausea would diminish after a few doses. I'm desperate for her to avoid a further fracture. Is there anything else that can protect her bones?*

A: I don't blame her for stopping a medication that gives her nausea at the age of 85. She is at an age when she is absolutely entitled to make that decision. There are alternatives. Another bisphosphonate would probably make her feel just as sick, so her doctor will probably prescribe strontium ranelate next, as one that has been shown to be reasonably well tolerated by older women. It doesn't produce as many side effects in the stomach and upper gut (such as indigestion, nausea and vomiting) as the bisphosphonates. However, around 6 per cent of women taking it have diarrhoea for the first few days, so she may be warned about that beforehand. Luckily, the loose stools are almost always a temporary inconvenience, and she should be able to continue with it.

# Useful addresses

There are many organizations dedicated to helping people with osteoporosis and to research into the disease. The **Arthritis Research Campaign, The National Osteoporosis Foundation** and **National Osteoporosis Society** are meant for doctors and researchers, but are open to anyone interested in developments in osteoporosis. They are, perhaps, heavy reading for people not trained in or familiar with medical jargon, but they contain well-researched and reviewed material and are the best, most up to date and most reliable websites on osteoporosis.

For people with a personal interest in osteoporosis

Information specifically provided by reputable societies can be found at the following, listed in alphabetical order, not necessarily in order of importance:

**Amarant Trust**
The Gainsborough Clinic
22 Barkham Terrace
80 Lambeth Road
London SE1 7PW
Tel.: 020 7401 3855
Helpline: 01293 413000 (11 a.m. to 6 p.m., Monday to Friday)
Website: www.amarantmenopausetrust.org.uk

This charity will help if you are interested in the use of HRT to protect yourself from osteoporosis. As its name suggests, its main aim is to help women with menopausal problems, but the doctors and nurses who run the helpline are fully aware of the needs of women with menopausal-related osteoporosis. The Trust also runs a not-for-profit self-referral menopausal clinic. You do not need a doctor's letter to attend it.

**Arthritis Research Campaign (ARC)**
Copeman House
St Mary's Court
St Mary's Gate
Chesterfield S41 7TD
Tel.: 01246 558033
Website: www.arc.org.uk

ARC was founded to finance research into all forms of arthritis, and osteoporosis comes into its remit as a considerable cause of backache. The organization offers booklets on back pain and its management.

103

**Family Doctor Publications**
Website: www.familydoctor.co.uk

Each booklet from this publisher is written by an expert doctor and they are all endorsed by the British Medical Association. Their series 'Understanding Illnesses' has an excellent booklet entitled *Understanding Osteoporosis*.

**The National Osteoporosis Foundation, USA**
Website: www.nof.org

A similar organization in the United States.

**National Osteoporosis Society**
Manor Farm
Skinners Hill
Camerton
Bath
Somerset BA2 0PJ
Tel.: 01761 471771
Helpline: 0845 450 0230
Website: www.nos.org.uk

The UK national osteoporosis charity, the aim of which is to eradicate osteoporosis and to promote bone health in men and women. The site provides useful information for the public, patients and health professionals. The Society encourages people to take action to protect their bones; the helpline is staffed by specially trained nurses; and it has a network of local support groups throughout the country.

**NHS Direct**
Tel.: 08457 90 90 90
Website: www.nhsdirect.nhs.uk

A wide range of information on osteoporosis, its prevention and treatment may be accessed from <www.nhsdirect.nhs.uk/en.asp?TopicID=340>.

For medical information and research

**The American Society for Bone and Mineral Research**
Website: www.asbmr.org

This society focuses on research in muscles and bones.

**The Cochrane Musculoskeletal Group**
Website: www.cochranemsk.org

The group reviews the evidence-based science behind osteoporosis research.

**The International Bone and Mineral Society**
Website: www.ibmsonline.org

There is a link from here to BoneKEy (<www.bonekey-ibms.org>), the only open-access online knowledge environment in the bone field. It is a fund of knowledge of the metabolism of bone, cartilage and minerals.

**The International Osteoporosis Foundation**
Website: www.iofbonehealth.org

Based in Canada, the foundation encompasses doctors, researchers, patient support groups, and pharmaceutical and other companies with an interest in osteoporosis. It also lists the addresses and websites for national osteoporosis societies around the world.

**Words of warning**
I have chosen the above websites and email addresses with care, as reliable sources of unbiased information. If you wish to surf the net looking for information on osteoporosis, be wary. Some websites have been set up by people with axes to grind, who have paid little attention to the need for scientific review of their opinions. Some of these sites are sponsored by commercial organizations with something to sell, or raise their revenue from advertising, which may make them biased towards their clients' products. I don't recommend them, so I am not listing any of them.

If you wish to know more about charities supporting osteoporosis, or for that matter any other medical charity, you will find what you need at the Charity Choice website (<www.charitychoice.co.uk>), and at the website of the Association of Medical Research Charities (<amrc.org.uk>).

# References

## 2 Bones – their structure and how they can go wrong

1 National Institutes of Health, 'Consensus development panel on optimal calcium intake: optimal calcium intake', *Journal of American Medical Association*, 1994, 272, pp. 1945–8.
2 Heaney, R. P. and Nordin, B. E., 'Calcium effects on phosphorus absorption', *Journal of the American College of Nutrition*, 2002, 21, pp. 239–44.
3 Lane, J. M. and colleagues, 'Osteoporosis: diagnosis and treatment', *Journal of Bone and Joint Surgery*, 1996, 78A, pp. 618–32.

## 3 Osteoporosis – the scale of the problem

1 Lippuner, K. and colleagues, 'Incidence and direct medical costs of hospitalization due to osteoporotic fractures in Switzerland', *Osteoporosis International*, 1997, 7(5), pp. 414–25.
2 Jordan, K. M. and Cooper, C., 'Best practice and research', *Clinical Rheumatology*, 2002, 15, pp. 795–806.
3 Freeman, K. B. and colleagues, 'Treatment of osteoporosis: are physicians missing an opportunity?' *Journal of Bone and Joint Surgery*, 2000, 82A, pp. 1063–70.
4 Kiebzak, G. M. and colleagues, 'Undertreatment of osteoporosis in men with hip fractures', *Archives of Internal Medicine*, 2002, 162, pp. 221–2.

## 4 Risk assessment and change

1 Woolf, A. D. and Akesson, K., 'Preventing fractures in elderly people', *British Medical Journal*, 2003, 327, pp. 89–95.
2 Ralston, S. and colleagues, 'Regulation of bone mass, bone loss and osteoclast activity by cannabinoid receptors', *Nature Medicine*, 2005, 11, pp. 774–9.

## 5 Making the diagnosis

1 Kanis, J. A. and Gluer, C. C., 'An update on the diagnosis and assessment of osteoporosis with densitometry', *Osteoporosis International*, 2000, 11, pp. 192–202.

2 Kanis, J. A. and colleagues, 'Clinical assessment of bone mass, quality and architecture', *Osteoporosis International*, 1999, 9, supplement 1, pp. 24–8.

## 6 The problems with fractures

1 Forsen, L. and colleagues, 'Survival after hip fracture', *Osteoporosis International*, 1999, 10, pp. 73–8.

## 7 Helping yourself (1) – supplements

1 The Record Trial Group, 'Oral vitamin D3 and calcium for secondary prevention of low-trauma fractures in elderly people', *The Lancet*, 2005, 365, pp. 1621–8.

2 Kitchin, B. and Morgan, S., 'Current opinion', *Rheumatology*, 2003, 15(4), pp. 476–80.

3 Reginster, J. Y. and colleagues, 'Influence of daily regimen calcium and vitamin D supplementation on parathyroid hormone secretion', *Calcified Tissue International*, 2002, 70, pp. 78–82.

4 Meyer, H. E. and colleagues, 'Can vitamin D supplementation reduce the risk of fracture in the elderly? A randomized controlled trial', *Journal of Bone Mineral Research*, 2002, 17, pp. 709–15.

5 Jensen, C. and colleagues, 'Long-term effects of nutrient intervention on markers of bone remodelling and calciotropic hormones in late-postmenopausal women', *American Journal of Clinical Nutrition*, 2000, 75, pp. 1114–20.

6 Wu, C. and colleagues, 'Epidemiological evidence of increased bone mineral density in habitual tea drinkers', *Archives of Internal Medicine*, 2002, 162, pp. 1001–6.

7 Sellmeyer, D. E. and colleagues, 'A high ratio of dietary animal protein to vegetable protein increases the rate of bone loss and the risk of fracture in postmenopausal women', *American Journal of Clinical Nutrition*, 2001, 73, pp. 118–22.

8 Dawson-Hughes, B. and Harris, S. S., 'Calcium intake influences the association of protein intake with rates of bone loss in elderly men and women', *American Journal of Clinical Nutrition*, 2002, 75, pp. 773–9.

9 Melhus, H. and colleagues, 'Excessive dietary intake of vitamin A is associated with reduced bone mineral density and increased risk for hip fracture', *Annals of Internal Medicine*, 1998, 129, pp. 770–8.

10 Feskanich, D. and colleagues, 'Vitamin A intake and hip fractures among postmenopausal women', *Journal of the American Medical Association*, 2002, 287, pp. 47–54.

11 Michaelsson, K. and colleagues, 'Serum retinol levels and the risk of fracture', *New England Journal of Medicine*, 2004, 348, pp. 287–94.

## 11 Today's medical treatments for osteoporosis

1 Bone, H. G. and colleagues, 'Dose-response relationships for alendronate treatment in osteoporotic elderly women', *Journal of Clinical Endocrinology and Metabolism*, 1997, 82, pp. 265–74.

2 Greenspan, S. L. and colleagues, 'Alendronate improves bone mineral density in elderly women with osteoporosis residing in long-term care facilities', *Annals of Internal Medicine*, 2002, 136, pp. 742–6.

3 McClung, M. R. and colleagues, 'Effect of risedronate on the risk of hip fracture in elderly women', *New England Journal of Medicine*, 2001, 344, pp. 333–40.

4 Gennare, C., 'Analgesic effect of calcitonin in osteoporosis', *Bone*, 2002, 30, supplement 5, pp. 67–70.

5 Chesnut, C. H. and colleagues (PROOF study group), 'A randomized trial of nasal spray salmon calcitonin in postmenopausal women with established osteoporosis: the prevent recurrence of osteoporotic fractures study', *American Journal of Medicine*, 2000, 109, pp. 267–76.

6 Neer, R. M. and colleagues, 'Effect of parathyroid hormone (1-34) on fractures and bone mineral density in postmenopausal women with osteoporosis', *New England Journal of Medicine*, 2001, 344, pp. 1434–41.

7 Body, J. J. and colleagues, 'A randomized double-blind trial to compare the efficacy of teriparatide with alendronate in postmenopausal women with osteoporosis', *Journal of Clinical Endocrinology and Metabolism*, 2002, 87, pp. 4528–35.

8 Black, D. M. and colleagues, 'The effects of parathyroid hormone and alendronate alone or in combination in postmenopausal osteoporosis', *New England Journal of Medicine*, 2003, 349, pp. 1207–15.

9 Finkelstein, J. S. and colleagues, 'The effects of parathyroid hormone and alendronate alone or both in men with osteoporosis', *New England Journal of Medicine*, 2003, 349, pp. 1216–26.

10 Meunier, P. J. and colleagues, 'The effects of strontium ranelate on the risk of vertebral fracture in women with postmenopausal osteoporosis', *New England Journal of Medicine*, 2004, 350, pp. 459–68.

11 Rizzoli, R. and colleagues, 'Presentation at the World Congress on Osteoporosis, 2004', *Osteoporosis International*, 2004, 15, supplement 1, p. 18.

12 Ettinger, B. and colleagues, 'Reduction of vertebral fracture risk in postmenopausal women with osteoporosis treated with raloxifene', *Journal of the American Medical Association*, 1999, 282, pp. 637–45.

13 Morello, K. C. and colleagues, 'Critical reviews', *Oncology and Hematology*, 2002, 43, pp. 63–76.

14 Royal College of Physicians of London and Bone and Tooth Society of Great Britain, *Osteoporosis: Clinical Guidelines for Prevention and Treatment*, London, Royal College of Physicians, 2000.

# 12 Hormone replacement therapy (HRT) – do you wish to take it?

1 Rossouw, J. E. and colleagues (Writing Group for the Women's Health Initiative Investigators), 'Risks and benefits of estrogen plus progestin in healthy postmenopausal women: principal results from the Women's Health Initiative randomized controlled trial', *Journal of the American Medical Association*, 2002, 288, pp. 321–33.

# 13 Non-drug treatments

1 Lieberman, I. H. and colleagues, 'Initial outcome and efficacy of "kyphoplasty" in the treatment of painful osteoporotic vertebral compression fractures', *Spine*, 2001, 26, pp. 1631–8.
2 Dudeney, S. and colleagues, 'Kyphoplasty in the treatment of osteolytic vertebral compression fractures as a result of multiple myeloma', *Journal of Clinical Oncology*, 2002, 20, pp. 2382–7.
3 Theodorou, D. J. and colleagues, 'Percutaneous balloon kyphoplasty for the correction of spinal deformity in painful vertebral body compression fractures', *Clinical Imaging*, 2002, 26, pp. 1–5.
4 Kannus, P. and colleagues, 'Prevention of hip fracture in elderly people with use of a hip protector', *New England Journal of Medicine*, 2000, 343, pp. 1506–13.
5 Cameron, I. D. and colleagues, 'Hip protectors improve falls self-efficacy', *Age and Ageing*, 2000, 29, pp. 57–62.
6 Wolf, S. L. and colleagues, 'Exercise training and subsequent falls among older persons', *Journal of the American Geriatric Society*, 1996, 44, pp. 489–97.
7 Iwamoto, J. and colleagues, 'Effect of exercise training and detraining on bone mineral density in postmenopausal women with osteoporosis', *Journal of Orthopaedic Science*, 2001, 6, pp. 128–32.

# 14 Future treatments

1 Jamal, S. and colleagues, 'Isosorbide mononitrate increases bone formation and decreases bone resorption in postmenopausal women', paper given at American Society for Bone and Mineral Research Annual Meeting, 27 September 2003.
2 Horwitz, M. J. and colleagues, 'Short-term, high-dose parathyroid hormone-related protein as a skeletal anabolic agent for the treatment of postmenopausal osteoporosis', *Journal of Clinical Endocrinology and Metabolism*, 2003, 88, pp. 569–75.

# Index